# FAT LOSS

# LOSS

## MANIFESTO

## SCOTT HAYWARD

# Fat Loss Manifesto

# Evidence Tracker

| Date | Total Weight | Lbs. FAT | Lbs. LBM |
|------|-------------|----------|----------|
|      |             |          |          |
|      |             |          |          |

Body Composition

## Calipers

| Date | Body Fat % | Bicep | Triceps | Back | Hip | |
|------|-----------|-------|---------|------|-----|---|
|      |           |       |         |      |     |   |
|      |           |       |         |      |     |   |
|      |           |       |         |      |     |   |
|      |           |       |         |      |     |   |

Inches

Notes:

| Date | Hips | Waist | Thigh | Upper Arm | Chest |
|------|------|-------|-------|-----------|-------|
|      |      |       |       |           |       |
|      |      |       |       |           |       |
|      |      |       |       |           |       |
|      |      |       |       |           |       |
|      |      |       |       |           |       |

*Goal Tracker*

The more often you see something in your mind's eye, the more quickly you'll reach it. The more intensely you see it, the more surely and completely you will attain it. Fill your mind with positive images. And soon your life will be filled with positive results.

| My Goal is…. | |
| --- | --- |
| My reason for this goal | |
| Steps I'll take | |
| Potential Obstacles | |
| Solutions to Obstacles | |
| Who will help me | |
| When I'll start | |
| When I'll meet my goal | |
| How I'll **reward** myself for making progress toward my goal | |

# Congratulations and Welcome
# to *THE* turning point in your life!

Imagine waking up 12-weeks from now, looking in the mirror and actually being amazed about what you see! You absolutely do have the ability to be in an entirely different body. From this moment on, you can expect that your mind, body and quality of life will only improve.

Making a commitment to follow the **Fat Loss Manifesto** guarantees the surest path to your ultimate fitness goals. In just 12 weeks, you will begin to see and feel dramatic changes with your body, and not just the obvious physical changes, you will also notice the psychological and physiological changes as well. Expect a decreased body fat percentage, increased lean muscle mass, increased metabolism, increased sense of well-being, an abundance of energy, lower bad and increased good cholesterol levels, decreased risk of heart disease, and the most important change of all… increased self-confidence.

Reaching your fitness goals will take effort and dedication. Throughout your transformation, you can depend on your Certified Fitness Professional to work with you every step of the way. You'll receive expert nutritional and fitness guidance, while being motivated and held accountable to stay focused as you progress through the program. However, it is important to realize that ultimately, only *you* have the ability to make sure you follow this program to the best of your ability in order to experience maximum results.

This Fitness Handbook is filled with the nut and bolts needed to achieve permanent fat loss. You'll discover dozens of helpful tips, motivational tactics and invaluable information allowing you to make informed decisions about nutrition, exercise and supplementation.

By following this complete, integrated program, along with the support of your Fitness Professional and your strong commitment to creating new and lasting habits for a fit and healthy lifestyle….**You can truly *Expect Success.***

# Introduction

**Fact:** There is no magic pill, special food or fat melting workout when it comes to fat loss and achieving the toned and sculpted body you desire.

There is one way to achieve permanent results; follow a complete and integrated fitness program that focuses on a change in **body composition** (body fat vs. lean muscle) rather than weight. It is lean muscle that plays the key role in any type of fitness program. Whether you're interested in fat loss or muscle gain, lean muscle requires certain conditions in order to allow a positive change in body composition.

## *Calories In vs. Calories Out*

To positively change the composition of your body (decrease fat, increase lean muscle) you have to know how to play the game of numbers. If you burn more calories than the calories you take in each day you will lose weight, this is called creating a caloric deficit. It is the *only* way to lose fat. If you do the opposite, take in more calories than what you burn, then you will gain weight.

Too much of anything gets stored as fat - even if you're eating nothing but healthy, supportive foods. If you eat too many of them, your body will still store the extra calories as fat. Even though this appears to be a simple concept, don't be fooled. The caloric deficit must be kept small for you want to maintain lean muscle and only lose fat weight. This strategy allows you to keep a high metabolism while at the same time transforming the shape of your body.

If calories are severely reduced, your body thinks you are starving and sets into motion a series of metabolic and hormonal events, which ultimately leads to muscle loss and a slower metabolism. Even more tragic, skipping meals and starving yourself causes your body to increase the level of fat storing enzymes so you are actually teaching your body to become efficient at storing fat!

## *Muscle is your Metabolism*

The amount of lean muscle you hold is directly related to your metabolism and your metabolism defines the shape of your body. Your metabolism is simply the rate at which your body burns calories. Lean muscle burns a lot more calories than fat so when you lose muscle, your metabolism drops and you burn fewer calories.

So not only must you take in sufficient calories to burn fat rather than muscle, it's also possible to build muscle, which in turn boosts metabolism. And the way to do this is, of course, to increase the amount of exercise you do. While aerobic activities such as running, swimming, fast walking help to tone muscle and burn extra calories, resistance training is the only way to increase the amount of muscle you have in your body. A consistent and effective exercise program is mandatory to help you to burn more calories and maintain or even build lean muscle mass. Your goal is to keep your activity up and your intake down and you ***will*** achieve results.

NOTE: It will be impossible to reach your best body by exercising more if you're neglecting nutrition. You won't get fit by eating supportively if you're missing workouts.

The **Fat Loss Manifesto** provides you with the complete formula for success:

## The Five Factors of Fat Loss
**Supportive Nutrition**
**Sensible Supplementation**
**Resistance Training**
**Smart Cardio**
**Personal Assistance**

Traditional fitness programs isolate only one or two factors. The truth is **all factors MUST be in place in order to bring about a lasting, positive physical change.** If any one factor is neglected or missing, the program will fail to produce results.

You are about to gain insight into exactly what you need to do and why you need to do it in order to achieve your ultimate fitness goals. Not only will your body transform, but you will also develop a better understanding how your body works. You will learn how to make wise, informed choices around a balanced nutrition and exercise program. In the process you will be able to replace unsupportive habits and develop a new outlook how to take complete control over how your body looks and feels and achieve a consistent, long-term fit and healthy lifestyle.

## Factor One: Supportive Nutrition

Nutrition has by far the greatest impact on fat loss. Eating supportively will not only allow you to improve your health and energy, and it also provides the ideal environment for your transformation - maintain lean muscle while reducing unwanted fat.

If your goal is to lose body fat, you must eat slightly fewer calories than you burn. This may seem simple, but when calories are reduced, the body becomes imbalanced. It is the body's job to restore balance, and it inevitably does so by either reducing the amount of calories it burns for energy ( by using muscle instead of fat) or by forcing you to eat more through hunger and cravings. This is one of the main reasons why fad diets do not produce long term results. The goal of our program is to ensure that you lose fat, not muscle.

Most fad diets are simply low-calorie diets disguised by great advertising or a clever marketing gimmick. There are currently thousands of diets listed with the Food and Drug Administration (FDA). This number alone proves that no one diet works long term. If a magic diet or formula for fat loss existed, everyone would be on it and no one would be overweight.

But why is it that some people do lose weight on diets? The immediate success most people experience from fad diets is due to water loss, eating fewer calories or a combination of the two. However, less than five percent of these dieters are able to keep the weight off. Diets simply don't work long term because of improper nutrition and the failure to change exercise and eating habits for life.

America is fatter as a society today because we consume approximately 300 to 500 more calories per day than we did 10 years ago, yet we move less because of advances in technology such as computers, escalators and other labor-saving devices.

Supportive nutrition can be mastered by understanding that everything you eat and drink can either positively or negatively affect your fat loss goals.

# Factor Two: Sensible Supplementation

Supplementation gives your body the nutrients it needs without adding calories. It is virtually impossible to satisfy your body's nutritional needs with the number of calories recommended to lose fat. In addition, due to a typically busy lifestyle, it is difficult to eat perfectly every day for the rest of your life. Therefore, when following a fitness program, muscles become undernourished, causing your body to shed the muscle it can't feed. By supplying the body with the natural nutrients it needs without additional calories, (e.g., whole food nutrient complex), you can help satisfy all your nutritional needs for repair and growth without exceeding the amount of calories your body needs to maintain the mandatory deficit for fat loss.

The benefits of using supplements as low-calorie nutrition during an exercise program are well researched. The daily use of a whole food nutrient complex has been found to be the most inexpensive nutritional insurance

The reason behind adding supplements to your daily meals is to supply the body with calorie-free nutrition and select, all natural compounds that have the potential to improve health, alter body composition and increase performance and metabolic rate.

## The Categories and Uses of Supplements

A whole food nutrient complex is the foundation of any complete fitness program. Additional vitamins, minerals, enzymes, essential fatty acids and antioxidants will boost your nutrient intake beyond what is available through the foods you eat. These additional nutrients allow cells to reach their potential creating the ideal environment for positive physical change. Taking other supplements before creating a nutritional foundation is like adding expensive accessories to a car that doesn't run properly.

<u>Altering Body Composition</u>
It is difficult to get enough nutrients from your normal diet to support your fitness goals. Any time there is an increase in cellular activity, as during exercise, the body increases its use of nutrients. By supplying these nutrients without additional calories, the attempt is made to satisfy all nutrient needs for repair and growth without exceeding the amount of calories needed to sustain the mandatory deficit for fat loss. When undernourished, the body must shed the muscle it cannot feed.

<u>Increasing Performance and Metabolism</u>
Specific nutrients and combinations of nutrients have been found to improve exercise performance and increase the calories burned during and after exercise. Supplying the body with calorie-free nutrients can improve performance and, therefore, assist with fat-loss and muscle-gain goals.

Sensible supplementation is highly recommended in order to supply the body with the right combination of calorie-free nutrients and compounds that have the potential to enhance performance, reduce body fat, increase muscle and improve health. Proper supplementation creates the environment your body needs to get maximum results.

# Factor Three: Resistance Training

Resistance training is the superior method of exercise for reshaping your body and shedding unwanted fat. Want to raise your metabolism? Start by understanding that the main tissue that burns calories is muscle, even at rest. Muscle is in essence, your fat burning machinery. The surest way to raise your metabolism and burn fat is to build and maintain muscle.

Resistance training is performed by using weights, machines and even your own body weight to effectively work your muscles. The goal of resistance training is to gradually and progressively overload your muscles so they grow stronger. This signals your body that it's growing and healthy, not deprived and starving.

As you increase your lean body mass, you increase your metabolic rate and this makes it easier to lose fat. With a faster metabolism, you'll burn more fat all day long - even while you're sleeping! Fat doesn't require any energy at all to maintain - it just sits there. That's why resistance training takes priority over cardio based exercise for people who want to lose body fat. Resistance training addresses the core of the problem – the rate at which the body uses energy, 24-7.

There are numerous reasons for increasing muscle beyond making clothes fit better. One of the major benefits is in the possible prevention and rehabilitation of bone injuries. Since proper resistance training strengthens the muscles as well as the supporting structures around the joint, this form of exercise will protect our joints from the stresses of an active lifestyle.

Another benefit of resistance training is improving the ability to perform daily activities. By increasing strength through resistance training, you move more efficiently with daily activities such as; lifting your children, carrying groceries, playing sports, moving furniture, taking out the trash etc.

The most important aspect of resistance training is correct performance of the exercise. Too many people become concerned with how fast an exercise is performed or how heavy a weight is being used. This means that the exercise is done incorrectly. This can cause injury and most often results in endless resistance training without benefit or results.

It is recommended that you commit to a full body resistance training program designed specifically for your body type, abilities and fitness goals for 20-45 minutes, at a minimum of 3 days per week. Allow at least one day of rest between workouts for muscle recovery and growth.

## The Benefits of Resistance Training

~ Increased Bone Density        ~ Improved Posture
~ Increased Lean Muscle Mass    ~ Improved Work Capacity
~ Increased Metabolism          ~ Reduces Depression
~ Increased Self-Esteem         ~ Increased Strength

# Factor Four: Smart Cardio

Cardiorespiratory exercise is a term that best describes the health and function of the heart, lungs and circulatory system. This system is considered the body's transportation network for it functions by circulating blood throughout the body. The goal of any cardio workout should be to get as many large muscles working as possible. They not only need to work hard, but continuously, in order to burn the greatest amount of calories during and after exercise.

**How much is too much? The Concept of "Smart Cardio":**
It is important to perform "smart cardio" for your body quickly adapts to cardio-based workouts. The more you do, the more efficient your body becomes, causing you to burn fewer calories from your fat stores each time you exercise.

Because your body adapts so quickly, cardio-lovers are forced to adjust their workouts to last increasingly longer in order to provide the same calorie burn. This not only increases the amount of time you have to spend in the gym but also increases the odds that your body may start breaking down muscle instead of fat for fuel.

Additionally, the benefits are temporary. Aerobic activity doesn't increase the amount of fat you burn after your workout like resistance training. Your metabolism returns to normal shortly after stepping off the treadmill.

Smart Cardio will greatly enhance the rate at which your body burns calories. The most effective Cardio programs are design around the **FITT Principles**: Frequency, Intensity, Time and Type.

## Frequency

Frequency refers to the number of times Cardio is performed per week. No less than three days per week, with no more than two days rest between workouts is recommended. For the first six weeks, beginners should work out every other day. However, if you are extremely overweight and perform a weight-bearing type of cardio (jogging, aerobic dance, etc.), rest at least 36 to 48 hours between sessions to prevent injury.

## Intensity

Intensity is described as the speed and/or the workload of a workout. When beginning a new exercise program, a Fitness Professional can determine the intensity level most appropriate and effective for you. It is important that you continually monitor the intensity level to ensure that you reach your fitness goals in the least amount of time.

There are many ways to effectively monitor exercise intensity. One common method is the talk test. The talk test means that at low to moderate intensity, you should be able to breathe comfortably and rhythmically throughout the entire workout. A good rule of thumb that's pretty effective is: If you are doing your aerobic exercise and are too out of breath to carry on a conversation, the odds are that you are working too hard. You need to back off a little. If, on the other hand, you feel as though you could just belt out your favorite song, you're probably not working hard enough. As long as you keep these two boundaries in mind, you'll probably be at the right intensity.

Another way to measure exercise intensity is with the use of a heart-rate monitor. A heart-rate monitor is considered the most accurate method of measuring pulse rate. If a heart rate monitor is unavailable, you can manually monitor heart rate by taking your pulse.

How to Take Your Pulse:

1. Place your index and middle finger on the inside of your wrist (about one inch from the top of wrist, on the thumb side).

2. Locate the artery by feeling for a pulse with the index and middle fingers. Apply light pressure to feel the pulse. Do not apply excessive pressure. It may distort your results.

3. When measuring the pulse at rest, count the number of times your heart beats in 60 seconds. Some factors that affect resting heart rate are digestion, mental activity, environmental temperature, biological rhythms, body position and cardiorespiratory fitness. As a result, resting heart rate should be measured immediately after waking or after you have rested for at least five minutes.

4. When measuring the pulse during exercise, count the number of beats in a six-second period and add a zero to that number.

Example: Number of beats in six seconds = 17. Add a zero = 170. Pulse rate = 170

Note: Use of the carotid artery in the neck is not recommended for measuring pulse rate. Pressure on the artery reduces blood flow to the brain, which can cause dizziness and an inaccurate measurement.

**Time**

Time is the length of time an exercise is performed, not including warm-up and cool-down. In order to gain Cardiorespiratory benefits, you may need to exercise for 20 to 30 minutes per session. It is important to remember that as you become more fit, both intensity and time can increase. You Fitness Professional will recommend when these adjustments should be made. Remember, more is not necessarily better.

**Type**

Type of refers to the activity used to create a stimulus. Before choosing an exercise, consider your goals, physical capacity, interests, available equipment and time constraints. Any activity that continuously uses larger muscle groups and is repetitive (rhythmic), in nature, is best.

*Treadmill Walking* (weight-bearing)

Walking is the most fundamental type of Cardiorespiratory activity. However, when performed on a treadmill, this simple exercise can become quite difficult for some participants. This difficulty may reside in the inability to maintain the necessary balance to perform the exercise properly and prevent injury. Maintaining balance involves controlling the position of the body's center of gravity. The center of gravity is the point around which the body balances. Therefore, when walking on a treadmill, focus on maintaining your center of gravity. Don't let your head move up and down, look straight ahead and keep your chest high to maintain balance and proper posture.

*Running* (weight-bearing)

Running is different than walking because of the additional impact it places on the body. Forces applied to the body while running are dramatic. Considering the fact that each foot strikes the ground 1500 times per mile, the potential for stress-related injuries significantly increases. To help prevent injury from overuse, gradually increase speed and/or distance. This will help your body adapt to the increase of force.

*Stationary Cycling* (non-weight bearing) Stationary bikes are another popular type of Cardiorespiratory exercise. Unlike walking or running on a treadmill, this non-weight bearing type of Cardiorespiratory exercise generally decreases the risk of injury. Before cycling, always adjust the seat height. Seat height is important because it influences the range of motion of the hip, knee and ankle while pedaling. The seat should be adjusted to match the standing height of the crotch. This will allow the knee to bend slightly at the bottom of the pedal stroke. Positioning of the feet is also important to consider while cycling. It is reported that the optimal foot position on the pedal is in the middle of the arch. Try to keep the force of the downward revolution in this area of the foot. When performed correctly, stationary cycling is considered a safe type of Cardiorespiratory activity.

*Elliptical Training* (low-weight bearing)

The word elliptical means shaped like an oval. The main difference with elliptical exercise machines is that although you are standing and bearing weight, which is important to building bone density, your feet never leave the footpads. So unlike treadmills or jogging, there is little impact on your joints and muscles. This provides a low impact, total body workout. The fluid, non-jarring motion makes the elliptical trainer ideal for anyone with back, knee, hips and joint problems. The dual action machines utilize both the legs and arm in providing a full upper and lower body workout.

*Jumping Rope* (weight bearing)

Jumping rope is an exercise we tend to overlook as adults. Jumping rope actually has a lot going for it as an exercise. Rope skipping can assist in developing agility, coordination, and balance, not to mention improvements in cardiovascular and muscular endurance. Because rope jumping is a fairly energetic exercise lots of calories can be burned during a twenty minute session of skipping. Current research is showing that high impact activities, such as jumping rope, can also help maintain and/or build healthy bones. Like all exercise programs, jumping for your health needs to be eased into. Jumping rope is a high impact, high intensity activity and those with health concerns should consult their physician before starting a jump rope program. As a coordination and agility builder, short bouts of jumping are sufficient. If you plan on using jumping rope as part of your aerobic routine, it's best to combine it with other aerobic activities, such as walking, biking, or running.

In the end, you want to make sure that your cardio is strengthening your heart and lungs and improving your cardio-respiratory efficiency, which is going to help oxygenate and feed every cell of your body. And you also want to make sure you're burning fat without sacrificing muscle tissue.

# Energy Expenditure Chart

The number of calories you burn depends upon your weight, the activity you are doing and the intensity level you are exercising at. Any activity you perform can be done at a variety of intensity levels. If you exercise at a higher intensity level, you will be working harder expending more energy and burning more calories than someone who is not working quite so hard. Remember that one pound of body fat is equal to 3500 calories. In order to lose one pound of fat you must burn at least 3500 calories! The following chart is a comparison of the average calories **burned per 30 minutes** of common activity per pound of body weight.

| Activity | 120 lbs. | 130 lbs. | 140 lbs. | 150 lbs. | 160 lbs. | 170 lbs. | 180 lbs. | 190 lbs. | 200 lbs. | 220 lbs. | 240 lbs. | 260 lbs. | 280 lbs. | 300 lbs |
|---|---|---|---|---|---|---|---|---|---|---|---|---|---|---|
| Aerobic dancing (low impact) | 138 | 149 | 161 | 172 | 184 | 195 | 207 | 218 | 230 | 253 | 276 | 299 | 322 | 345 |
| Aerobics step training, 4" (beginner) | 174 | 189 | 203 | 218 | 232 | 247 | 261 | 276 | 290 | 319 | 348 | 377 | 406 | 435 |
| Backpacking with 10 lb. Load | 216 | 234 | 252 | 270 | 288 | 306 | 324 | 342 | 360 | 396 | 432 | 268 | 504 | 540 |
| Basketball (game) | 264 | 286 | 308 | 330 | 352 | 374 | 396 | 418 | 440 | 484 | 528 | 572 | 616 | 660 |
| Basketball (leisurely, nongame) | 156 | 169 | 182 | 195 | 208 | 221 | 234 | 247 | 260 | 286 | 312 | 338 | 364 | 390 |
| Bicycling 10 mph (6 min/mile) | 150 | 162 | 175 | 188 | 200 | 213 | 225 | 237 | 250 | 275 | 300 | 325 | 350 | 375 |
| Bowling | 66 | 72 | 77 | 82 | 88 | 94 | 99 | 105 | 110 | 121 | 132 | 143 | 154 | 165 |
| Cross country snow skiing, leisurely | 186 | 202 | 217 | 232 | 248 | 263 | 279 | 294 | 310 | 341 | 372 | 403 | 434 | 465 |
| Gardening (moderate) | 108 | 117 | 126 | 135 | 144 | 153 | 162 | 171 | 180 | 198 | 216 | 234 | 252 | 270 |
| Golfing (walking , w/o cart) | 120 | 130 | 140 | 150 | 160 | 170 | 180 | 190 | 200 | 220 | 240 | 260 | 280 | 300 |
| Golfing (with a cart) | 84 | 91 | 98 | 105 | 112 | 119 | 126 | 133 | 140 | 154 | 168 | 182 | 196 | 210 |
| Hiking, no load | 186 | 202 | 217 | 232 | 248 | 263 | 279 | 294 | 310 | 341 | 372 | 403 | 434 | 465 |
| Housework | 108 | 117 | 126 | 135 | 144 | 153 | 162 | 171 | 180 | 198 | 216 | 234 | 252 | 270 |
| Ironing | 60 | 65 | 70 | 75 | 80 | 85 | 90 | 95 | 100 | 110 | 120 | 130 | 140 | 150 |
| Jogging, 5 mph (12 minutes/mile) | 222 | 240 | 259 | 278 | 296 | 315 | 333 | 352 | 370 | 407 | 444 | 481 | 518 | 555 |
| Raking | 90 | 98 | 105 | 112 | 120 | 128 | 135 | 142 | 150 | 165 | 180 | 195 | 210 | 225 |
| Running, 08 mph (7.5 minutes/mile) | 366 | 396 | 427 | 458 | 488 | 518 | 549 | 579 | 610 | 371 | 732 | 793 | 854 | 915 |
| Running, 10 mph (6 minutes/mile) | 420 | 455 | 490 | 525 | 560 | 595 | 630 | 665 | 700 | 770 | 840 | 910 | 980 | ## |
| Skipping rope | 342 | 370 | 399 | 428 | 456 | 484 | 513 | 541 | 570 | 627 | 684 | 741 | 798 | 855 |
| Snow shoveling | 234 | 253 | 273 | 292 | 312 | 332 | 351 | 371 | 390 | 429 | 468 | 507 | 546 | 585 |
| Soccer | 234 | 253 | 273 | 292 | 312 | 332 | 351 | 371 | 390 | 429 | 468 | 507 | 546 | 585 |
| Stair climber machine | 192 | 208 | 224 | 240 | 256 | 272 | 288 | 304 | 320 | 352 | 384 | 416 | 448 | 480 |
| Swimming (25yds/minute) | 144 | 156 | 168 | 180 | 192 | 204 | 216 | 228 | 240 | 264 | 468 | 312 | 336 | 360 |
| Tennis | 192 | 208 | 224 | 240 | 256 | 272 | 288 | 304 | 320 | 352 | 384 | 416 | 448 | 480 |
| Vacuuming | 90 | 98 | 105 | 112 | 120 | 128 | 135 | 142 | 150 | 165 | 336 | 195 | 210 | 225 |
| Volleyball (game) | 144 | 156 | 168 | 180 | 192 | 204 | 216 | 228 | 240 | 264 | 288 | 312 | 336 | 360 |
| Walking 2mph (30 minutes/mile) | 72 | 78 | 84 | 90 | 96 | 102 | 108 | 114 | 120 | 132 | 144 | 156 | 168 | 180 |
| Walking 3mph (20 minutes/mile) | 96 | 104 | 112 | 120 | 128 | 136 | 144 | 152 | 160 | 176 | 192 | 208 | 224 | 240 |
| Walking 4mph (15 minutes/mile) | 120 | 130 | 140 | 150 | 160 | 170 | 180 | 190 | 200 | 220 | 240 | 260 | 280 | 300 |
| Weeding | 120 | 130 | 140 | 150 | 160 | 170 | 180 | 190 | 200 | 220 | 240 | 260 | 280 | 300 |
| Weight training (40 sec. Between sets) | 306 | 332 | 357 | 382 | 408 | 433 | 459 | 484 | 510 | 561 | 612 | 663 | 714 | 765 |
| Weight training (60 sec. Between sets) | 228 | 247 | 266 | 285 | 304 | 323 | 342 | 361 | 380 | 418 | 456 | 494 | 532 | 570 |
| Weight training (90 sec. Between sets) | 150 | 162 | 175 | 188 | 200 | 213 | 225 | 237 | 250 | 275 | 300 | 325 | 350 | 375 |

# Factor Five: Personal Assistance

The more customized your program is for you, the better your results will be. When you combine an effective fitness program with proper nutrition, supplementation and accountability, you can make incredible changes.

It is the job of your Fitness Professional to give you the right amount and type of work for your goal and ability. However, your body is naturally driven to adapt to this workload (i.e. plateau). A plateau occurs when the body adjusts to changes in internal and/or external conditions or circumstances. Science is still unable to predict when a person will plateau, but one thing is for certain – it will happen..

Doing the same type of exercise without variation or failing to increase the challenge when your body "adapts" to the present workload, are just two examples of conditions that will steer your results to a complete halt. In order to avoid a plateau during your transformation, your Fitness Professional will make changes in your exercise routine or eating habits to help you reach the next level. The best way is not to do more of the same, but try new exercises or change the frequency, intensity, or duration of the routine.

Even though your Fitness Professional individualizes each of the components necessary to begin the journey toward your goal, it does not end there. There are many factors that may affect when and how significantly the other four components will need to be manipulated to keep you on the path to success. Your Fitness Professional will help you avoid plateaus by keeping your body in a caloric deficit (adaptation period) until you look the way you want. This can only be accomplished by following all 5 Components and correctly applying the information provided in this fitness handbook.

## What to Expect

Over the next several weeks, you will meet in a small group setting with your Fitness Professional. Together you will work with all 5 Factors of Fat Loss during each session to improve your ability to achieve and maintain your fitness goals.

## Program Overview:

**Session One:** Establishing a Starting Point
        Topic: Body Composition and Setting Goals

**Session Two:** Record Keeping and Portion Sizes
        Topic: Using a Food Log to Develop Awareness and Control

**Session Three:** Your Supportive Nutrition Plan
        Topic: When, What, How – Building your Menu

**Session Four:** Meal Management Strategies
        Topic: How to Plan for Success

**Session Five:** Super Charge your Nutrition Plan
        Topic: A Well Nourished Body Burns More Fat

**Session Six:** Reassessment
        <u>Topic:</u> Reflect and Reassess Goals

**Session Seven:** Food Labels 101
        <u>Topic:</u> Become a Label Detective

**Session Eight:** Healthy Fast Food
        <u>Topic:</u> How to Make Informed Choices

**Session Nine:** Master your Motivation
        <u>Topic:</u> Maintain it and Move Forward

**Session Ten:** Plateau Busters
        <u>Topic:</u> Specific Steps to Create Change

**Session Eleven:** Conquer Self-Sabotage
        <u>Topic:</u> Create Positive Beliefs; Create Positive Outcomes

**Session Twelve:** New Beginnings
        <u>Topic:</u> Final Assessment and Long-Term Strategies

# How to Make the Most of Each Session

One of the secrets to achieving successful results is the use of Reflection. Just as we use a mirror to improve our outward appearance, we can also use the power of reflection as a tool that will improve us from the inside – in our minds and behaviors. At the end of each lesson, you will find a Reflection Log to write about what you have read or learned in class, with the goal of transforming that experience into knowledge that can be used in all future situations.

You are essentially creating an action plan. As you read through each lesson and participate in each class, you may come up with an idea, thought or approach that can be assimilated into your lifestyle to create a positive change. Take a moment to highlight it or write it down. Do it while it's fresh in your mind. Use this handbook as your guide to develop your TO DO list of strategies and ideas for each week. This will help to hold you accountable so you TAKE ACTION to implement the ideas. Make them real. Make them happen.

Make a commitment to yourself to study this handbook for 10 minutes a day. That's all it will take to assimilate the information. Use your Reflection logs each day to write down your ideas for taking action. Then IMPLEMENT! The secret to your success is RAPID, INCREMENTAL INTEGRATION of what you learn. That means you need to be implementing bits and pieces of what you learn each and every day. But take it one session at a time. Don't make your TO DO LIST overwhelming. If you do, you'll just become frustrated and discouraged and revert back to old, unsupportive habits. Be realistic. Give yourself time to absorb all of this new information but begin the process of implementation TODAY!

# Personal Commitment Contract

At this time, we would like you to make an executive decision and pledge your full commitment to this program. Our goal is to provide you with the necessary information to make the appropriate steps toward a healthier lifestyle. Ultimately, **you are responsible** for your own results. To be successful, you must dedicate one or more of the following attributes.

| | | |
|---|---|---|
| ~ Effort | ~ Critical thinking | ~ Commitment |
| ~ Honesty | ~ Consistency | ~ Enjoyment of the process |

With this contract, you will promise to satisfy all of the necessary commitments to help you reach your health and fitness goals. Commit to this program like you would any high-importance task at work or at home and commit to getting the most from the program.

### REWRITE the Personal Commitment Contract in the spaces provided below.

I, _____, promise to commit to the (course name) program to the best of my abilities by looking at myself and my life honestly, thoroughly
and without judgment for the next ten weeks.
I promise that before I skip any of the assignments or disregard advice, I will sit
down and re-read this contract.
I promise to remember the **REASONS** I am doing this program, especially when I
am tempted to stop.
I promise to recognize the inevitable negative feelings and frustrations which
may come up for me during the program , while recognizing and honoring them as my
feelings, will not empower them by allowing them to stop me.

_____
_____
_____
_____
_____
_____
_____
_____
_____
_____
_____
_____
_____
_____
_____
_____
_____
_____
_____
_____
_____

_____   _____
Signature                                    Date

# The 12-Week Solution

It's not enough to eat supportive foods and exercise for only a few weeks or even a couple months. You must incorporate these behaviors into your life to achieve lasting results. Lifestyle changes start with taking an honest look at your eating habits and daily routine.

When you combine the Five Factors of Fat Loss, you take total control of that word we talked about earlier… metabolism. And it is your metabolism that defines the composition of your body. As you begin to change the way you eat and move, your appetite will change, your energy levels will change and then you will find, in a very short time, that if you go more than three hours without eating or skip your regularly scheduled workout, you will be affected!

You've made it clear that you're not happy living in the body that you are in. It's time to take responsibility for creating the body you desire. You have to start creating new habits.

This may be quite a change for some, and change is not always easy. Our promise to you is that if you apply the Five Factors of Fat Loss and make the commitment for just one week, and really stick with it, you will find it very difficult to go back to your old way of living.

**The Power of Habit**
Success and failure are simply habits, and the good news is that good habits are just as difficult to break as bad ones. Motivation gets us started on the road to success and good habits are the fuel that keeps us making progress. Just as bad habits can lead to a downward spiral, good habits escalate and lead to an upward spiral.

Welcome the challenges that face you. With effort and patience you have the full potential to create a positive change with your physique and your quality of life. There are only three conditions necessary for the acquisition of any new habit or skill. The COURAGE to try something you do not know how to do, the PATIENCE to try again once you have discovered that you don't know how to do it and the PERSEVERANCE to keep trying, as many times as necessary, until you do know how to do it.

**What You Will Notice – The Benefits**
The first thing most people inevitably notice when they apply the Five Factors of Fat Loss is a dramatic change in their energy level. You will wake up in the morning and be surprised that you actually have energy!

As you put quality fuel into your body – regularly – and when you optimize the way your body functions through a combination of smart cardio and resistance training, you will start to appreciate what energy REALLY is!

When you change your habits and apply a formula that guarantees results, you will begin to feel a change in your energy levels as quickly as three to four days. So, within a couple of weeks, typically, you will probably start noticing your clothing fits differently – perhaps a little looser. That doesn't mean you should jump on the scale if weight loss is a goal. You will soon discover why the scale is EVIL. It can't tell the difference between water weight, adipose (stored body fat) weight, and muscle weight. So, when your clothes start to feel looser, realize that something good is happening. Fat is leaving your body.

As you change your habits and consistently apply the Five Factors of Fat Loss, others will notice a change before you ever do. Someone who hasn't seen you in a couple weeks may suddenly say "Wow! You look great?" You can count on the next question they'll ask to be something like, "Are you on a diet?" And you can quickly reply "No! I'm just eating more and exercising less." You will leave them feeling stunned! But eventually they'll ask you how you did it – and they may end up applying the same factors themselves!

## Guarantee your Success

Before you begin this life-changing journey, you must accept and live by the basic understanding that this course is built around the premise of "progress, not perfection." By developing awareness that improvement is measured by your daily progress, you can save yourself a lot of grief and frustration from the get go. Simply focusing on small, positive steps in everything you do is a vital component to a permanent physical change. With time, commitment and a willingness to continue to take those small steps, failure is not an option.

The following steps will ensure that you receive the maximum benefit from your experiences. They will play an essential role in helping you achieve your goals of ultimate leanness and energy. Improvement will become apparent in a matter of weeks.

## I will...

1. **Decide on what I want to achieve** – Have a clear vision of the end result. Close your eyes and visualize your ideal body. Picture exactly how you look, size and shape you are and how you feel.

2. **Know and feel my REASON** for wanting to achieve these particular results – Continue to ask yourself "why" until you elicit an emotional response.

3. **Believe I am capable and deserving** of reaching this goal – If others can do it, why can't you?

4. **Make this a priority** in my life, every day – "We do not set out to fail, we simply fail to plan" - Schedule workouts, schedule your meals, keep kitchen stocked…

5. **Start taking actions** that bring results – each day strive to do something a little better than the day before. "I am making progress if I am better today than I was yesterday" ~Dr. Wayne Dyer.

6. **Be grateful** - understand that the quickest way to achieve my goals is to be happy NOW. When you look to the future for your happiness, you can guarantee you'll never be happy. Focus on the present. Life shouldn't be something to be endured until the future arrives. Your present should be thrilling, exhilarating and inspiring.

7. **Be forgiving** - I will not beat myself up when I haven't done everything perfectly. If I slip, I will quickly return to my plan. I won't feel guilty, but will remain enthusiastic about the process and with myself.

You can begin, right now, by taking a different, more positive course of action. Allow this handbook to be your guide as you strengthen your commitment. Take a chance, have faith and proceed with confidence. You are about to become yet another success story; joining hundreds who have successfully learned how to eat, how to move and how to believe in themselves once again. They are experiencing the joy of living life to the fullest. So will you.

# Session One: Establishing a Starting Point

To individualize your Program, a starting point must be determined. During your initial one-on-one consultation, your Fitness Professional will assesses your current body composition and eating habits to determine your initial statistics and provide basic recommendations. Your health, fitness level and lifestyle habits are determined from the Client Profile Packet.

## Body Composition

The shape of your body is determined by three things: muscle, bone and fat. While there's really nothing you can do about changing your bone structure, there is a whole lot you can do about muscle and fat. This ratio of muscle to fat is commonly known as your body composition. To determine a beginning body composition value, your Fitness Professional will measure body fat percentage, circumference measurements and weight.

It is important to realize that altered body composition is attained through fat loss and lean muscle tissue gain, **not weight loss**. When your body receives the proper amount of calories and nutrients, you can reach and maintain your fitness goals. Additionally eating supportive foods that fuel muscle tissue will help burn fat efficiently during exercise and when at rest.

**Why is it important to understand the difference between fat loss and weight loss?**

> ➤ Calories are burned in muscle tissue. One pound of lean muscle burns approximately 50 calories a day. Conversely, body fat is a store house for calories. One pound of fat burns approximately 5 calories a day and stores 3500 calories of energy.
> ➤ By simply restricting calories to shrink the number on the scale, a minimum of 25% of weight loss (more than two pounds per week on average) will be lost from lean tissue.
> ➤ As a result, your metabolism will be suppressed by 50%.
> ➤ Rapid weight loss from under-eating causes muscle tissue to be used for energy, which cripples your body's ability to burn fat for energy. In the future this will cause you to put the weight back on and most likely gain more than you ever had before.
> ➤ Providing your body with a regular exercise program and the food and nutrients it needs will sufficiently fuel working muscles, initiate fat loss and develop an accelerated, fat burning metabolism.
> ➤ Proper fat loss strategies will allow you to lose 75% of your weight from fat and less that 25% from lean tissue.

## Calorie Estimation

Under eating or overeating may cause muscle tissue loss or fat gain. In order to reach your goals, both you and your Nutritional Coach need to know the amount of food you eat. One way to do that is to use a calorie estimation equation.

---

**Men:** RMR= 293 – 3.8(age) + (456.4 x height in meters) + (10.12 x weight in kg)
**Women:** RMR= 247 – (2.67 x age) + (401.5 x height in meters) + (8.6 x weight in kg)
1in = 0.0254 meters
1kg= 2.2lbs

---

If you know the lean body mass number from the body fat calculation then use that number as the weight in kg.

**RMR in Weight Loss program:**

**RMR x 0.85:** 1-1.5# weight loss per week
**RMR x 1.0:** 0.5-.75# weight loss per week
**RMR x 1.3:** 0-0.5# weight loss per week
**RMR x 1.4-1.6:** weight maintenance for most people
**RMR x 1.6-1.9:** weight maintenance for moderately active people
**RMR x 1.9-2.5:** weight maintenance for very active people (athletes)

Once you have determined your Resting Metabolic Rate (RMR) then multiply that number by the number set according to the goal that is listed next to it. This will be your estimated calories you will need to consume consistently every day. Re-evaluate this every 3-4 weeks because as your weight drops you will need less calories. Also, not every person is the same so the calculation may say one number, but you need to lower the calories or increase your exercise level to actually get in a calorie deficit and start lose weight.

**How to lose body fat instead of muscle tissue:**

- Make positive changes in your daily eating habits
- Adhere to your supportive nutrition plan
- Commit to at least 3 days of resistance training and cardio.
- Take at least 10,000 steps a day (GET A PEDOMETER)
- Eat about one to two hours prior to exercising to fuel muscles and prevent muscle loss
- Have a recovery drink within 30-45 minutes after exercise to replenish nutrients in muscle tissue and expedite recovery
- Take a whole food nutrient complex that is specifically designed for you to prevent muscle tissue loss. This in turn boosts your metabolism.

## How do you measure Progress?

Weight, body composition and circumference measurements are only a few of the many tools used to gather **evidence of your progress**. They should not, however, be thought of as the only way to measure success. There are several methods for measuring your progress. Our approach uses simple strategies to help keep you focused but at the same time – avoiding frustration.

**CLOTHING:** Find evidence by taking a trip to your very own closet. Take out a pair of pants that fit snugly before you began your new, healthy habits. Are you able to ease into them, when before you had to sit (or lie) down and yank them up your legs? This is a sure sign of progress toward a leaner you! Jeans are actually the best form of measurement because they are the least forgiving. They just won't stretch to fit in those bulging areas. They will be your benchmark for you well you are progressing through this course. Try them on every 3-4 weeks. Unlike the scale, jeans do NOT lie. They can't. They are ALWAYS the same size.

**BODY MEASURES:** Other numerical signs of progress. Watch the measurements of your waist, arms, neck and hips change. If you are not losing pounds, are losing inches all over your body as your figure slims down and tones up. Other numerical indicators include a reduction of blood pressure or cholesterol, BMI, and body fat percentage.

**ENERGY LEVELS:** Monitor how a eating supportively and regular exercise affects your energy levels. Not only will you be able to work out for longer intervals of time, but daily movements and chores will also become easier. Whether cutting the grass or simply walking up the stairs, these behaviors will come effortlessly. Think of all the daily activities you could use more energy for—grocery shopping, house cleaning, playing with your kids, and more. Pretty soon you'll be training for your first 5K!

**EMOTIONALLY:** Lastly, be conscious of how you feel emotionally. You work hard to reach your goals. Hopefully, the hard work will come with a boost in self-esteem, confidence, and happiness. Are you beginning to feel more comfortable in your own body? What do you hear others saying to you? What are you saying to yourself?

## Setting Healthy Goals

The first step to achieving results is setting a realistic goal. No matter what the reason, successful and healthy weight management depends on sensible goals and expectations. If you set sensible goals for yourself, chances are you'll be more likely to meet them and have a better chance of managing your weight long term.

Setting healthy goals at the start of an ongoing program can help you change and improve your physical activity and eating habits. To set goals that are right for you, think about what you want to change and why, and what steps you can take to reach your goal. These changes don't have to be big. Even small steps can make a difference. Also, think about who can help you, and how you'll reward yourself for making these changes.

### 5 Steps to Setting Goals

**Make a choice** - Look at your body, your quality of life. What do you really want to have?
**Be specific** - Leave no detail left behind.
**Find Your Reason** – Now that you know what you want to change, ask yourself WHY?
**Form your plan** – What is it going to take to get there? What are you going to have to do?
**Take action** - Do you know what the number one cause of failure is in most people's lives? Never taking action. We develop these comfort zones and become afraid to step out of those boundaries and really go after our goals. We know that we must change; we know that we have to follow our plan to be happy, but seldom do. Do not let your written plan of action go to waste. Start immediately on working towards your goals!

Your Fitness Professional will guide you in completing your Goal Tracker Sheet during session one. Realistic expectations are based on the fact that – safe and long term weight loss is 1-2 pounds of fat per week, 2-3 months to drop one size or 2 inches off a belt size.

---

## Complete...

All actions start with a change -- no matter how small. This is the first step toward making that change: an inventory of exactly how you really feel about losing weight and exactly what you are willing (and in many cases, not willing) to do.

1. List 3 Things you want to change about your body.

2. Why is this so important to you? What is your Reason?

3. IDENTIFY: List the habits or actions that have contributed to why your body is the way it is today. (What are you doing right now that allows you to keep this body?)

4. List 3 things you could do right now that will make a difference today (an action, no matter how small, that will bring you closer to your goal).

5. List at least 2 things that you are giving up by not being more fit or having a body you can be happy in. What is it costing you? (If you're really ambitious and want some extra credit, try tackling this one as well: What do you gain by keeping things the way they are? What's the hidden payoff?)

**Write in your Fitness Journal for at least 3 days. Be as specific and consistent as possible. You will share your findings during our next class.**

# Session Two: Record Keeping and Portion Sizes

**Do you know how MUCH you are eating?**
One of the key ways to promote fat loss is to control your portion sizes. Research has shown that Americans often underestimate how many calories they are consuming each day by as much as 25%. If you are a healthy eater, it is possible to sabotage your efforts by eating more than the recommended amount of food. If nutrients are available at proper times and in the proper quantities, your body can use them for energy to keep you feeling full, promote muscle growth and burn fat.

**Importance of accuracy**
Under eating or overeating may cause muscle tissue loss or fat gain. A serving isn't what you happen to put on your plate. It's a specific amount of food defined by common measurements, such as cups, ounces or pieces.

**How to Estimate Portion Sizes**
Learn food weights, measurements and portions by using the examples below and by using a food scale, measuring cups and spoons in your kitchen.

Typical Portion Sizes:

- 1 ounce of cheese is about the size of 4 dice
- 1 fruit serving is about the size of a baseball
- 1 serving (½ cup) of vegetables, pasta or rice ½ of a baseball
- 3 ounces of cooked meat, fish, or poultry is about the size of a deck of cards
- 2 tablespoons of peanut butter is about the size of a large marshmallow
- 1 serving (1 cup) of milk, yogurt or fresh chopped greens is a fist

**Tips:**

- Take time to "eyeball" the serving sizes of your favorite foods.
- Measure out single servings onto your plates and bowls, and remember what they look like.
- Avoid serving food "family style." Prepare plates with appropriate portions in the kitchen, and don't go back for seconds.
- Never eat out of the bag or carton.

**What gets Measured, Gets Managed**
One of the most powerful ways you learn is from yourself, keeping a journal will teach you more about you than any book you read or course you take. Many people are unaware of their unsupportive habits. Denial and vague ideas are of no use in the process of achieving results. You need to be in control of the way you eat and move and all the variables and you can't control something you've never measured! ENTER – The Fitness Journal

Your goal is to keep a journal for at least 3 days. You get to choose three days that are a typical representation of your general eating and exercise habits (one work day, one training day, and one weekend day, for example) and on those days record everything you eat and the workouts that you perform. There are two reasons do this as soon as you get started.

One, you need to see how "off" your nutrition is. Two, you to see how "off" your nutrition is. Even if you don't record your foods accurately, you'll have to make a conscious choice to guess or omit – which is an admission to yourself (though not to your Fitness Professional) that your nutrition and exercise habits need improvement.

It is inevitable that there will be some of you who are simply lazy and forget to record, while still others are so deep in denial that they'll lie outright with no regrets. For both types, sticking to an integrated fitness program will be either extremely difficult or impossible. For most people, journals are excellent motivational tool and will help them commit to new, supportive habits.

**FYI:** Tracking your daily food intake and exercise habits is a great way to take action and prove to yourself that you are serious about your achieving your goals! Don't worry about the occasional setback – you are only human! Instead of giving up entirely, simply start fresh the next day. Make an effort to do better than you did the day before. Keep in mind that lifestyle changes won't happen overnight. Be patient, make small changes and gradually add new supportive habits.

### Journal Guidelines:

**Time:** Write the time of day you ate the food.

**What kind:** Write down the type of food you ate. Be as specific as you can. Don't the "extras," such as soda pop, salad dressing, mayonnaise, butter, sour cream, sugar and ketchup.

**How much:** Record the amount and calories of the particular food item you ate.

**Where:** Write what room or part of the house you were in when you ate. If you ate in a restaurant, fast-food chain or your car, write that location down.

### Helpful Hints:

1. Be Honest. There's nothing to be gained by trying to look good in your journal. Your Fit Pro can help only if you record what you really eat.
2. Record what you eat each day. Keep your journal with you all day, and write down everything you eat or drink.
3. Do it now. Don't depend on your memory at the end of the day. Record your eating as you go. Be Specific. Make sure you include "extras," such as gravy on your meat or cheese on your vegetables.

**By keeping records of your past, you will shape your future. See something you like in your past? Work to replicate it. See something you don't like? Work to re-shape it.**

# Portions, Weights, Measures and Conversions

| Dry Measures | | Liquid Measures |
|---|---|---|
| 3 tsp. | 1 Tbs. | ½ fl. Oz |
| 6 tsp. | 2 Tbs. | 1 fl. Oz |
| 4 Tbs. | 1/4 cup | 2 fl. Oz. |
| 5 1/3 Tbs. | 1/3 cup | 2.7 fl. Oz. |
| 8 Tbs. | 1/2 cup | 4 fl. Oz. |
| 12 Tbs. | 3/4 cup | 6 fl. Oz. |
| 16 Tbs. | 1 cup | 8 fl. Oz. |
| 2 cups | 1 pint | 16 fl. Oz. |
| 4 cups | 1 quart | 32 fl. Oz. |
| 4 quarts | 1 gallon | 128 fl. Oz. |

## Volume Measures

| | | |
|---|---|---|
| 1 tsp. | 1/3 Tbs. | 1/6 fl. Oz. |
| 3 tsp. | 1 Tbs. | ½ fl. Oz. |
| 2 Tbs. | 1/8 cup | 1 fl. Oz. |
| 4 Tbs. | ¼ cup | 2 fl. Oz. |
| 5 ½ Tbs. | 1/3 cup | 2 2/3 fl. Oz. |
| 8 Tbs. | ½ cup | 4 fl. Oz. |
| 10 2/3 Tbs. | 2/3 cup | 5 1/3 fl. Oz. |
| 12 Tbs. | ¾ cup | 6 fl. Oz. |
| 14 Tbs. | 7/8 cup | 7 fl. Oz. |
| 16 Tbs. | 1 cup | 8 fl. Oz. |

Many foods increase in volume when they are cooked. Compare the dry and cooked measures of the following foods.

| Food | Dry Measure | Cooked Measure |
|---|---|---|
| Barley | 1 cup | 3 ½ cups |
| Beans, dried | 1 cup | 2 cups |
| Buckwheat/Kasha | 1 cup | 2 ½ cups |
| Bulger Wheat | 1 cup | 2 ½ cups |
| Cornmeal | 1 cup | 3 cups |
| Lentils | 1 cup | 2 ¼ cups |
| Lima, baby | 1 cup | 1 ¾ cups |
| Lima, regular | 1 cup | 1 ¼ cups |
| Noodles | 8 oz. Dry | 4 cups |
| Oatmeal | 8 oz. Dry | |
| Pasta | | |
|     Cooked firm | 8 oz. Dry | 4 ¼ cups |
|     Cooked soft | 8 oz. Dry | 5 ¼ cups |
| Couscous | 1 cup | 2 cups |
| Rice | 1 cup | 3 cups |
| Rice, wild | 1 cup | 3 ½ cups |
| Whole wheat, grains/berries | 1 cup | 2 2/3 cups |

# Your Guide to Food Serving Sizes

## Carbohydrates: Bread, Cereal, Rice & Pasta Group: (80kcal/serving)

**1 Carbohydrate serving =**

| | |
|---|---|
| 1 slice of bread | ½ cup flaked cereal |
| 1oz of ready to eat cereal | ½ cup of cooked cereal |
| ½ cup of cooked rice or pasta | ½ bagel (3.5") |
| ½ large baked potato | 1/3 cup couscous |
| ½ cup corn | ½ cup peas |
| ¼ cup baked beans | 1/3 cup kidney beans |
| 2 taco shells (6in) | 3 cups of cooked popcorn |
| 6 saltines | 1 slice of angel food cake |
| 1 biscuit | ½ hot dog or hamburger bun |
| 1 cup clam chowder | 3 small fat-free cookies |
| 2" piece of corn bread | 1 corn on the cob |
| 3 graham crackers | 6 butter crackers |
| 1 dinner roll | ½ english muffin |
| 1 small muffin | 1 small pancake |
| 3 cups popped popcorn | ½ pita |
| 3 hard pretzels | 10 pretzel sticks |
| 2 rice cakes | 4 ounces spaghetti sauce |
| 2 pieces of licorice | ½ cup yams |
| 1 granola bar | 5 animal crackers |
| 1 small waffle | 3 fig newtons |
| 3/4 cereal bar | ½ cup stuffing |
| ½ cup mashed potatoes | 2 rice cakes |
| ¼ large bagel (4.5") | 2 Bread Sticks 4in long |
| 1 Pita 6 in across | 1/4c granola |
| 1 flour Tortilla 7-8 in across | 1/4c grape nuts |
| 1 ½ cups puffed cereal | ½ c sugar frosted cereal |
| 1 tablespoon honey | 1 Fruit snack (1 roll) |
| ½ Acorn Squash | ½ cup cooked barley |
| ½ medium sweet potato | 1 cup butternut squash |
| ¼ cup hummus | 1 medium white potato |
| ½ large whole wheat pita | |

## Vegetable Group: (25kcal/serving)

**1 Vegetable serving =**

| | |
|---|---|
| 1 cup of raw leafy vegetables | 1 cup tomato juice |
| Artichoke, 1 small | 1 cup zucchinii |
| 1 cup of V-8 juice | ¾ cup bean sprouts |
| ½ cup steamed broccoli    1cup raw | 1cup eggplant |
| 1 cup steamed cabbage, 2 cups raw | 5 raw mushrooms |
| ¼ chopped onion | ½ cup green beans |
| 1 cup yellow squash | 1 cup asparagus, 10 spears |
| 1/3c boiled beets | 1c cooked/raw cauliflower |
| ½ cup steamed greens (collards, kale) | ½ cup steamed okra |
| ½ cup raw green, yellow, red peppers | 1 med tomato |
| 2 cups raw turnips | ½ cup salsa |

**Vegetables that can be eaten in unlimited quantity**
Celery, cucumber, lettuce, radish, and watercress

## Fruit Group: (60kcal/serving)

**1 Fruit serving =**

| | |
|---|---|
| 1 medium size piece of fruit such | ½ cup of canned fruit |
| as an apple, banana, or orange, peach, pear | ½ cup of chopped raw |
| ¼ cup of dried fruit | fruit |
| ½ cup of apple juice | ½ cup of applesauce |

| | |
|---|---|
| 8 halves of dried apricots | 12 fresh cherries |
| ¾ cup canned grapefruit | ½ cup of pears |
| 3 teaspoons jelly preserves | ½ cup fruit salad |
| 1avocado | ¾ cup blueberries |
| ½ cup grapes | 1 fig bar |
| 2 medium plums | 3/4 cup pineapple |
| 2 Tbsp raisins | ½ cup fruit cocktail |
| 1cup honey dew melon | 2 Kiwi |
| ¾ cup mandarin oranges | 1 ¼ cup watermelon |
| 1cup raspberries | ½ cup orange juice |
| ½ cup grapefruit juice | 1/3 cup prune juice |
| 2 small nectarines | 4 med apricots |
| 1 cup blackberries | ½ med cantaloupe |
| ¾ whole mango | 2cups watermelon chunks |

## Milk, Yogurt, & Cheese Group: (90-150kcal/serving)

**1 Dairy serving =**

| | |
|---|---|
| 1 cup of milk (skim, 1%, 2%) | 1.5 oz of natural cheese |
| 1 cup of plain yogurt | ½ cup of evaporated |
| 2 ounces of mozzarella cheese | skim milk |
| 1cup nonfat cottage cheese | ¾ 2% cottage cheese |

## Protein: Meat, Poultry, Fish, Dry Beans, Eggs & Nuts Group: (35-100kcal/serving)

**1 Protein serving =**

| Low Fat | Medium Fat | High Fat |
|---|---|---|
| 1 ounces of fish | 1 ounce ground round or ground chuck | 1 ounce of beef |
| 1 ounce shellfish | ¼ cup tofu | 1 ounce ham |
| ¼ cup of egg substitute | | 1 tablespoon peanut butter |
| 1 ounce chicken | | 1 ounce of nuts |
| 1 ounce turkey | | 2 sausage links |
| 2 egg whites | | |
| 1 ounce shrimp or tuna fish | | |

### Vegetable Protein + 1 Starch

| | |
|---|---|
| ½ cup of black beans | ½ cup cooked red beans |
| ½ cup cooked kidney beans | ½ cup cooked lentils |
| ½ cup black eyed peas | 1/3 cup cooked soy beans |
| ½ cup cooked white beans | ½ cup cooked garbanzo bean |
| ¾ cup cooked green peas | |

## Fats: (45kcal/serving)

**1 Fat serving =**

| | |
|---|---|
| 1 tsp oil (canola, olive, peanut) | 8 large olives |
| 1 tsp margarine | 1tsp mayonnaise |
| 1 Tbsp reduced fat mayonnaise | 1 Tbsp salad dressing |
| 1 Tbsp cream cheese | 2 Tbsp sour cream |
| 1 tsp butter | 6 whole small walnuts |
| 1 Tbsp Sunflower seeds | ½ Tbsp Almond butter |
| 1 tsp Flax oil | 6 whole small pecans |
| 6 whole small cashews | 1/8 med avocado |
| ½ Tbsp cashew butter | |

# Session Three: Your Supportive Nutrition Plan

Making supportive food choices is your secret weapon in the quest to achieve a toned and sculpted body. Eating supportive foods frequently will help you lose fat and increase your energy dramatically.

## The Basics of Supportive Nutrition

Macronutrients are nutrients that provide calories or energy. All food (protein, carbohydrates and fats) can be used for energy. Not only does your body need all three for growth, metabolism, and for other body functions, the *quality* of these nutrients contribute to satiety and are broken down at different rates. The "thermic effect of food" the energy your body uses to digest food, accounts for *10 percent* of your daily calorie burn. This has a powerful affect on your body's ability to lose fat. When it comes to nutrition for Fat Loss, your goal is to INCREASE the calories burned by eating multiple, highly thermic meals.

## Protein
- Protein provides four calories per gram. Thermic Effect: for every 100 cal = 20 cal are burned
- Besides water, protein is the most plentiful substance in the body. Made up of structural units or chains called amino acids

### What does it do?
- In the absence of sufficient carbohydrates, protein is used as an energy source.
- Protein is the primary component of building material for muscles, blood, skin, hair and internal organs such as the heart and the brain. Used in the formation of hormones, enzymes and antibodies
- Protein is vital for growth, maintenance and repair of body tissue.

### Sources of protein:
- Complete Proteins: Complete proteins contain all the essential amino acids (not made by the body) Sources include: Animal products such as beef, chicken, fish, milk and cheese.
- Incomplete Proteins: Incomplete proteins do not contain the adequate of essential amino acids. Sources include: Plant products such as grains, legumes, cereals, nuts and starchy vegetables.

## Carbohydrate
- Carbohydrates provide four calories per gram. Thermic Effect: for every 100 cal = 10 cal are burned

### What does it do?
- Your body's main source of fuel
- Carbohydrates are converted to glucose (blood sugar), your body's primary energy source.
- Glucose is used to help burn fat for a fuel.

### Sources of carbohydrates:
- Complex: Complex carbohydrates have larger chains of sugars (starches) that must be broken down before being absorbed into the body and utilized for energy or stored. Complex carbohydrates *require more energy* to digest. Sources include: starchy vegetables, fibrous fruits, whole grain pasta, bread, cereals and crackers.
- Simple: A simple carbohydrate contains one or two sugar molecules that are easily absorbed into the body and used for energy in the form of glucose (blood sugar) or stored for future use (fat). Sources include: table sugar, honey, cola drinks, juices, candy, cakes, etc.
        ********* SIMPLE CARBOHYDRATES have NO Thermic Effect**************

## Fat
- Fat provides nine calories per gram. Thermic Effect: for every 100 cal = 5 cal are burned
- There are three classifications of fats
    1. <u>Saturated fats</u> -found in animal sources (accept coconut and palm oil) and are solid at room temperature (lard or the fat on steak). They are a source of cholesterol.
    2. <u>Trans fats</u> also called hydrogenated fats have no physical purpose in your body. These fats are made when foods are processed, found in just about everything that has been boxed or changed from its natural state. Common sources are cakes, muffins, chips, crackers, doughnuts and popcorn.

3. <u>Unsaturated fats</u>: these fats are primarily found in plant sources, are liquid at room temperature (olive oil). These are the healthy fats.

**What does it do?**
- Fat provides energy for aerobic energy metabolism (sitting, walking, jogging)
- Fat assists in membrane cell structure, function and hormone production
- Fat transports and mobilized fat soluble vitamins in the body.
- Fat contributes to satiety

**Sources of Fat:**
- Saturated sources: meats such as ribs, chicken with skin, dairy foods, butter, most fast food, etc.
- Unsaturated sources: salad dressing, oil, margarine, mayonnaise, nuts, avocados, fish oil, etc.

## What am I supposed to eat?

So what determines which sort of weight you will lose? The types of foods that you eat along with how big of a caloric deficit you create will be the main factors in determining your body's ability shed fat. A supportive nutrition plan includes whole foods: lean proteins, whole grains, fruits, veggies and healthy fats. Specific examples are provided in the Supportive Menu Chart.

Each time you eat, your body must expend some energy to digest food. Each type of food creates different demands for energy expenditure - Thermic Effect of Food. This is what sets each of these nutrients apart and divide them into smaller versions to absorb them into your bloodstream to perform a variety of tasks – some are used to help burn fat and build muscle.

When foods are processed, much of this work is done for you. For example, processed flour is ground into small pieces that the body can digest more quickly. This means your blood sugar rises faster and your body expends fewer calories processing the flour. Whole foods, on the other hand, pack more nutrients, are higher in fiber, and force the body to work harder to use them as energy.

## Meal timing

Consuming food triggers digestion, and digestion requires calories. By eating more frequent, smaller meals, you continuously supply your body with nutrients while forcing it to digest and break down the foods. This, in turn, can have the net effect of raising your metabolism.

Ideally, you want to eat a supportive meal every 3 hours. Eating frequently stabilizes your blood sugar levels, providing a steady flow of quality fuel to your muscles and brain. This helps to steady your mood and boost your energy. Besides making you feel better, this increased energy can help further fat loss because you will naturally want to be more active. Another benefit of a stable blood sugar levels is a suppressed appetite. By eating a supportive meal, frequently, you are reprogramming your appetite. You will begin to have fewer cravings and binge less often because you no longer experience the pain of hunger.

When you constantly give your body food with small meals your body does not feel the need to store fat. On the contrary when eating large, infrequent meals your body feels the need to store some food as fat for it is unsure as to when it will be fed again.

Eating frequently throughout the day can also help you stay energized and avoid making poor food choices. Eating smaller balanced meals often helps to reduce blood sugar fluctuations and leads to stronger compliance in making supportive food choices and long term success.

**Skipping meals** will only sabotage compliance. Missing a normally scheduled meal will leave you hungry, increasing the likelihood of making a poor food choice. As the day wears on, lack of proper meal timing will most likely cause you to become so hungry that you will forget about sticking to a supportive nutrition plan. It then becomes a matter of eating anything to satisfy your hunger!

## Eating Fewer Calories

To lose fat you **have** to eat – not starve yourself. The only way that the human body burns off body fat is by being in caloric deficit. The goal is to adjust your daily calorie intake slightly to initiate fat loss. Restricting your calories *will* allow you to experience weight-loss, but it will be the result of muscle loss. When this occurs, not only does the body burn muscle to fuel its energy requirements, but by ridding itself of muscle, you are essentially slowing your metabolism.

**NOTE:** To reduce body fat, a useful guideline for creating a caloric deficit is to reduce your calories by at least 500, but not more than 1000 below your maintenance level. For people with only a small amount of weight to lose, 1000 kcal will be too much of a deficit. As a guide to minimum calorie intake, the American College of Sports Medicine (ACSM) recommends that calorie levels never drop below 1200 calories per day for women or 1800 kcal per day for men. Even these calorie levels are very low and put you at risk for loss of muscle and a lower metabolism.

## The Formula

You will not receive an individualized menu or the perfect calorie count. Two reasons: first there is no "magic" number. One of the main problems with diet programs today is that they over-emphasize the numbers. Yes, food is fuel, but food should also be pleasurable. It is simply not realistic if every time you needed to eat you had to calculate and weigh your food, you would give up. Eating supportively should not become a chore. This is why we integrated the concept of the **Supportive Menu Chart**. It is much easier to look at your plate and notice that you have a lean protein, a starchy carbohydrates and a fibrous carbohydrates.

Secondly, we could create the perfect menu plan, but you won't follow it – at least not the majority of the time. This was our protocol in the past. Our Fitness Professionals would spend hours creating the perfect menu plans for clients. But time after time, clients reported their frustration and inability to follow such an idealistic menu plan. However, these same clients experienced amazing results.

Our conclusion; as long as you make an effort to change the way you eat each and every day, no matter how small the change, you will achieve results.

## The Balance

For those of you who need the numbers, you can figure out what percentage of your meal should be protein, carbohydrates and fat. The numbers here can only be very general and educated guesses. You are going to have to do some trial and error to see what is best for you.

These are numbers based upon averages, based upon what tends to work for most people. You may find that you'll have to change it around just a little bit.

> Of the calories in each meal, <u>approximately</u>:
> - 60% from carbohydrates
> - 25% from lean proteins
> - 15% from fats (with as little of that as possible coming from saturated and hydrogenated sources)

**Cheat Meals!**

Everyone loves to indulge in Cheat Meals. Simply having something to look forward to is extremely motivational. It makes it much easier to avoid temptation in the short term. On the other hand, the fundamentals of successful fat loss remain constant...If you make a point of eating cheat meals often enough, you reduce the chances of successful fat loss.

As you apply these supportive nutrition habits, you make your body very efficient at burning through calories. And then, on occasion, you can put a not-so-supportive into your body because it is going to be quite good at burning through it. You're going to enjoy that favorite food even more, because it's become a special treat.

**A general rule on cheating**: make sure that no more than 10% of your meals are missed or cheat meals. So if you're eating six meals a day, seven days a week (for a total of 42 meals per week), then no more than four of those meals should be misses or cheats. If you can achieve 90% adherence you will without a doubt get the results you want.

---

## Complete...

1. What is the Thermic Effect of Food?

2. Which nutrient has the highest Thermic Effect? Why?

3. Create a highly thermic meal using the Supportive Menu Design chart.

4. How does the consumption of Sugar prevent Fat Loss?

5. Why are Cheat Meals beneficial? Describe how you will plan your Cheat Meals.

# Session Four: Meal Management Strategies

Skip breakfast? Eat your heaviest meals at night? You're only setting yourself up for failure. In order to achieve your goals you must develop and practice meal management strategies.

**Plan To Succeed**
Having a plan is essential if you are truly serious about creating a positive physical change. Obviously it takes a good amount of planning, preparation, and persistence to get into the habit of eating this supportively and this frequently. You must prepare your food well ahead of time. Initially it will be a bit tedious, but once you get into the habit you'll see some amazing changes.

Plus, when meals are balanced and timed appropriately, you can avoid energy swings and non-productive food choices. Modern lifestyles in our fast-paced world have made it difficult to prepare a food plan for a week, much less a day.

## TIMING
**BREAKFAST** - The most important meal of the day. If you are someone who thinks skipping breakfast will help you lose weight, think again! Studies have shown that those who skip breakfast are 4 ½ more likely to be obese than those who don't.

The average 8 hours of sleep burns about 450 calories, therefore your body needs to refuel within 60 to 90 minutes of waking. Eating breakfast is like adding kindling to the fire of your metabolism.

If you skip breakfast, your metabolism slows down and your blood sugar drops. As a result, you become hungry, have less energy and your body will be more likely to store fat. You are just setting yourself up to impulsively snack in the morning - often on high-fat sweets - or to make up for those lost calories by eating extra servings or larger portions later in the day.

Need more proof? A recent study conducted by the National Weight Control Registry at the University of Colorado found that those who had lost and maintained at least 30 pounds for at least one year ate breakfast every single morning.

**Eat Every Two to Three Hours.**
Eating once or twice a day is a sure fire way to lose muscle and lower your metabolism. As you already know, less muscle mass and a lower metabolism is not the way to get to your goal. To control your appetite, regulate your blood sugar level and build lean muscle mass, you must eat every 2 – 3 hours.

Understanding how your body's blood sugar levels rise and fall explains why you need to continually refuel your body. Normally when you eat, your blood sugar, or glucose levels, will rise, level out, and then drop in about three hours. If you don't eat again within three hours or so, your blood sugar begins to drop even further. If your blood sugar drops too low, your body starts kicking in an emergency mechanism to make sure there's enough sugar around for brain, heart and other organ function. It does this by "catabolizing" lean muscle mass. In other words, your body starts eating your muscle for energy. This will only slow down your metabolism; you'll burn the muscle you're trying to build which sabotages your body's ability to burn fat.

Eating five to six meals a day also provides your body with the energy it needs to contend with daily activities and stress. Digesting food requires energy, which cranks up your metabolism. So the more frequently you eat, the more calories you burn. The bottom line is you'll maintain consistent energy levels and turn your body into an efficient, fat burning machine.

### Pre and Post Workout Fuel

If you're spending time exercising and putting energy into your workouts, it only makes sense that you eat the right foods before and after your workouts if you really want to reach your goals. Yet many people exercise on an empty stomach and fail to refuel after a workout.

### Fuel your Workout

By not eating, your body uses muscle protein for fuel because it doesn't have enough carbohydrates to burn. If you start your workout well-fueled, your body will burn a combination of the carbohydrates stored in your muscles and the fat stored in your fat cells.

Ask yourself how many times have you stopped exercising because you felt dizzy, shaky, or just plain tired? That's because you didn't have enough fuel to go the distance. Have a small meal of composed of complex carbohydrates about an hour before your workout. A Prograde meal replacement shake is a great alternative if you are pressed for time or do not like the heavy feeling of working out with a "meal" on your stomach. You will have the energy to workout with the intensity necessary to maximize the results of your workout and you'll avoid experiencing low blood sugar jitters and dizziness.

### Replenish your Muscles

It's important to make the right choices after you exercise. Otherwise, your hard work won't yield the results you want. After a workout, your body's energy levels are considerably depleted and must be replenished.

Eating a properly balanced meal 30 to 45 minutes after your workout does two important things. One, it helps your body to recover quickly, which is needed for muscle growth because of tissue repairs and for replacing lost glycogen in the muscles. And two, it helps muscle growth.

A liquid meal replacement shake such as Prograde Varsity has the perfect balance of carbohydrate and proteins that can be quickly absorbed. Drinking your post workout meal is an excellent strategy. Not only are liquids easily digested and absorbed at a faster rate, but after exercising there is a window of about an hour when your ability to absorb nutrients is exceptionally high. After that time your uptake of nutrients returns to normal, so don't miss the opportunity to feed your hungry muscles.

When you help your body recover from the stress imposed upon it (exercise) by ingesting the proper nutrients at the right time, the quicker you will be able to affect body composition change (gain muscle, lose fat or both). You will automatically help your body "bounce back" and you will see results in less time.

# BALANCING
## Give Your Body What it Needs.

Eating a meal that is balanced to include carbohydrates, proteins and fats gives your body everything it needs to function efficiently and feel its best.

CARBOHYDRATES: The main fuel source. Carbohydrates supply your body with energy. Without an adequate supply of carbohydrates, your body goes into carbohydrate deprivation. This is called a state of ketosis (your body is using protein "muscle" as energy). This is not good to be in for very long because it will rob your body of muscle tissue in an effort to create energy.

Carbohydrates come in two forms: simple and complex. Simple carbohydrates are for quick energy like fruit juice. Complex carbohydrates are used for timed-released and lasting energy. Fruits, vegetables and whole grains are good sources of complex carbohydrates and make you feel more satisfied after a meal.

PROTEIN: The building blocks of muscle. Next to water, protein is the most abundant material in the human body. While consuming enough protein is essential for growth and development of the body, eating huge amounts will not build muscle. In order to build muscle, protein must be consumed with enough carbohydrate calories to provide the body with energy. It's important to eat the right amount and the right kind of protein to get the results you want. Choose lean cuts of meat, fish, low fat milk, nuts, beans or soy products.

FATS: The most misunderstood nutrient. Your body needs fats to manufacture hormones, for proper brain function and for healthy joint lubrication. In addition, fats release energy slowly, providing a necessary feeling of fullness by prolonging digestion. Eliminate fats completely from your diet and watch your energy/strength levels go down as well as your sex drive. Also your skin will get dry and your hair will lose its shine. Be sure to eat healthy, unsaturated fats. Look for them in nuts, fish oils and seeds. Ensure your daily fat intake by supplementing with Prograde's EFA Icon. It is very common in western society today to consume foods that are low or even deficient in essential fatty acids. In fact, the typical diet contains too much Omega 6 fatty acids and not enough Omega 3. When there is too much Omega 6 fats this promotes the production of inflammation causing chemicals in the body. Fortunately, EFA Icon is a powerful source of the potent Omega 3 fatty acids your body craves for optimal health. In fact, the unique formulation in Prograde EFA Icon of Antioxidants, Neptune Krill and Omega 3 fatty acids enhances cellular function, decreases inflammation, and improves body composition, health and well-being.

Each meal should contain a portion of each of the macronutrients. Eating the recommended balance creates a favorable environment that leads to muscle growth, fat loss and optimal health.

## Go for Variety

Eating a variety of foods is the untold secret of "happy" weight management. According to several studies, those who had difficulty adopting a nutrition plan ate the same foods week in and week out. Don't make the same mistake! Before you sit down to plan your menus and make out your grocery list, plan to include at least one new food a day or week.

When you think about variety, think about eating the full rainbow assortment of fresh fruits and vegetables on a regular basis. If you use this tactic, you won't become bored and tempted to choose high-calorie snacks and you'll improve your nutritional intake at the same time

## Bonus Fat Loss Rule:

Go to bed early and get adequate rest every night. Two reasons: Lack of sleep increases the hormone *cortisol,* which is a hormone that stores fat and burns muscle (in other words, it does the exact opposite of what you are trying to accomplish), and decreases your testosterone levels (which need to be high in order to keep your fat burning/muscle gaining processes going at full speed). While sleep requirements vary, seven to nine hours of sleep is generally a good rule of thumb. The probability of succumbing to late night cravings increases exponentially for every late hour of the day that you stay awake.

# PLANNING

## Supportive Menu Design

Take the time to plan when, where and what you will eat. Set aside a few minutes each week to think about the meals you'll need for the upcoming week. Begin by creating an outline, based on your lifestyle, showing when you will eat each day (approximate times) and how you will fit a supportive meal into every 2 –3 hours. Once you have a plan, create a variety of meal options. Keep it simple in the beginning. It should only take a few minutes to lay out 7 breakfast meals, 7 lunch meals, 7 dinner meals, and 2-3 additional snacks for each day. Then ask yourself two questions. (1) Which foods do I need from the store to make these meals? (2) What foods do I already have in the house? Make your shopping list from your answers to these questions.

## Pack your Lunch

One thing that totally kills a sound nutrition plan is going to work. Work, however, is not the culprit. The culprit is Lunch Hour. If you do not pre-pack your meal, lunch comes along and you will end up going to the nearest fast food joint and exposing yourself to temptation. Therefore, the best way to stay on your nutrition plan (and also avoid losing meals) is to pre-pack everything in such a way that when a meal time comes, it is relatively easy to have access to the food.

## Cook in Bulk

After a long, hard day at work, the last thing you probably feel like doing is going home to slave over a hot stove to cook a meal. Whether you cook for yourself or prepare meals for your family, you know how much time it takes to prepare and get food ready each and every day. And you already know that eating at restaurants may be convenient, but they're not an ideal option if you're trying to eat supportively, as meals out can be high in calories and have poor nutrient profiles.

The best way to reduce the tedious time spent preparing meals and still stick to a healthy eating plan is to pick one day per week to plan and prepare your meals and snacks for the entire week. That way, you don't need to worry about cooking every night. All it takes is a couple of hours of planning, and cooking can be one fewer thing that you'll have to worry about in your busy day.

Keep your meal strategy simple by cooking a lot of supportive, easy to cook food (i.e. chicken breast, steamed vegetables, brown rice, etc.) one day per week. Begin with your menu plan. Be easy on yourself and plan at least three of the five meals that use the same food as a main ingredient. Measure out and divide up your daily meals into Tupperware containers for individual storage.

All it takes is a little planning and a dedicated day once a week to get your plan on track. Cooking and preparing foods shouldn't be a time-consuming hassle. By planning your week and preparing your foods ahead of time, you won't have to rely on takeout food or make unhealthy choices at the end of your busy day.

## Be Prepared with Portable Snacks

How many times this past week have you eaten on the run? No place is safe either – the car, your desk, maybe even the shower! Your time is strapped, your body is tired, and you need food that's easy to grab 'n' go. It is very easy to forget eating healthy.

Make your own supportive snacks portable and easy for on-the-go eating. Prepared ahead of time, they can be tossed into a gym bag or purse.

- Celery sticks with peanut butter and raisins
- Whole wheat crackers with peanut butter
- Low-fat cheese cubes
- Hardboiled eggs
- Trail mix
- Vegetable sticks with a packet of low-fat dip
- Yogurt and granola
- Box of raisins or other dried fruit
- Apples, bananas, strawberries and a handful of nuts
- Whole-wheat crackers and low-fat string cheese
- Fruit smoothie in a thermos
- Tuna and cottage cheese in mini-containers

## Make a Shopping List

Grocery stores are very tempting places. They are carefully designed by experts to persuade you to buy. So unless you know what you are looking for, you can easily end up buying a ton of items you didn't plan for. Before stepping foot in the grocery store, plan out what types and amounts of foods you will eat throughout the week by making a shopping list. This will help you to comply with your nutrition plan.

Never shop for groceries on an empty stomach. Hunger increases temptation. If you are hungry when you shop for food, you will be led astray.

Shop the outside aisles. Grocery stores are designed with the four basic food groups on and around the perimeter. If you stick to the outside aisles, you'll find produce, bakery, dairy and meat -- the most natural, unprocessed foods which are best for your health. Avoid going up and down the aisles where processed "convenience" foods dwell to tempt you away from healthy foods.

# Complete...

1. Plan four portable, supportive snacks that you would eat during the week.

## 2. Take Inventory

Your environment supports your habits. If there's nothing bad in the house to eat, chances are you're going to eat properly. Take a moment to survey what items you have in your pantry and refrigerator. What can be discarded? What can be replaced?

3. Why is it important to eat every 3 hours?

4. List 3 ways to minimize temptation the next time you go to the grocery store.

# Session Five: Super Charge your Nutrition Plan

**FACT:  Nothing burns fat better than healthy muscles.**
A healthy human body is made up of over 50% lean muscle…..over 600 muscles! Muscle not only defines the way your body looks, it controls your metabolic rate.

In your quest to realize your fitness goals, it's common to lose focus on the real things that really matter, such as your health and well-being. Thus, you end up neglecting your overall state of health. Cutting down on your daily calorie intake does not necessarily assure a effective fat loss.

When your muscles are not properly cared for through consistent, effective exercise or if they are undernourished, your muscles will deteriorate. When that happens, you will gain fat and your health begins to fail.

**How do you properly care for your muscles?**
The best way to get the most nutrients is to combine supportive, nutrient-rich whole food sources; "super foods" with a whole food nutrient complex such as Prograde's VGF+25. Both sources have a direct impact on the overall health of your body and at the same time will optimize your fat burning ability when combined with an effective workout program.

VGF+25 provides your body with the nutrients naturally found in whole foods. These are the nutrients your body was designed to use in order to heal, promote and maintain optimum health. The cells of your body were intended to absorb and be nourished by natural food. Because your body recognizes VGF+25 as food, nutrients are readily absorbed and utilized for nourishment and balance.

Here's a quote from a special report put out in 2006 by the Harvard Medical School's School of Public Health: "Diet alone cannot provide everything. It's difficult to get enough of certain nutrients from food." Fact: In order to obtain the full spectrum of vitamins and mineral, you would have to eat about 5,000 calories a day.

**So Do You Really Need to take a Supplement? Absolutely!** It's no longer a question! A whole food supplement will fill a lot of holes that if left empty will hinder your body's ability to burn fat efficiently. Supplements compensate for important nutrients the average American diet often lacks This is particularly important when attempting to lose body fat. The balanced nutrition provided by VGF+25 helps stabilize your body's chemistry, raising your metabolism and increasing your body's ability to absorb vital nutrients – all without added calories! Sensible supplementation promotes fat loss without losing muscle by supplying the essential nutrients necessary to increase or maintain lean muscle tissue.

The Result: Your body is more prepared to fight illnesses and has the raw materials necessary to achieve a lean, fit physique.

In a perfect world, we would eat perfectly balanced meals that contain just the right amount of each vitamin that we need for optimal health and well being without adding calories that lead to weight gain. Whole food supplements serve as buffers in the event that your diet does not meet your daily requirements. At the very least, a whole food nutrient complex such as Prograde's VGF+25 is insurance against unavoidable dietary shortcomings no matter how you eat.

## The Nutrients you Need for Optimum Health and Fitness

Did you know there are 45 known essential nutrients (nutrients must come from outside, sources) 13 kinds of vitamins, and at least 20 kinds of minerals that are required in specific amounts for the body to function properly?

## Macro and Micronutrients

| Macronutrients (have calories) | Micronutrients (do not have calories) |
|---|---|
| Proteins | Vitamins |
| Carbohydrates | Minerals |
| Fats | Water |

Vitamins and minerals are simply catalysts that allow metabolic processes to take place. Vitamins and minerals act on the macronutrients you take in – the proteins, carbs and fats in your diet. So if you're not taking in a balanced diet of proteins, carbs and fats, the vitamins and minerals can't do their job.

## Enzymes

Enzymes are required for your body to function properly. Without enzymes you wouldn't be able to breathe, swallow, drink, eat, or digest your food. You must have enzymes to help perform these tasks. Each metabolic reaction is started, controlled, and terminated by enzymes. Without enzymes, no metabolic activity will occur.

When you were young, you had an abundant supply of enzymes. You felt great. Your energy level seemed never ending. You had "enzymes to burn" which kept you running at tip top efficiency. Over the years as you eat overcooked and processed foods, you are using up your natural supply of digestive enzymes. So, as you age, digestion becomes more difficult for your body. The reason we are running out of enzymes is a LIFESTYLE PROBLEM. Our poor dietary habits, fast food obsessions, and excessive intake of fat and sugars, all require excessive amounts of enzymes to digest our foods.

## Amino Acids

Amino Acids are the "building blocks" of the body that make up proteins. Protein substances make up the muscles, tendons, organs, glands, nails, and hair. Growth, repair and maintenance of all cells are dependent upon them. Next to water, protein makes up the greatest portion of our body weight. A deficiency in even one of the 20 will severely compromise your health.

## Essential Fatty Acids (EFA's)

Essential meaning your body can't live without them. These are the "good" fats needed for a heart health, a healthy nervous system, and especially a healthy brain (the human brain is around 80% fat). Protein alone does not build muscle. EFA's are the starting point - or the mortar and brick - for manufacturing all other fatty acids and hormones necessary to build strong lean muscle while increasing stamina required for building lean muscle EFA's Aslo helps to decrease inflammation and pain; reduced muscle soreness after strenuous workouts and shortened recovery time

**Phytonutrients "Antioxidants"**

Antioxidants are cell protectors. They protect cells from the damage caused by unstable molecules known as *free radicals*; the devils that roam around your blood stream, causing damage to cell walls. Free radicals also accelerate the aging process. Also, over a long time period, such damage can become irreversible and lead to diseases like cancer. Antioxidants interact with and stabilize free radicals and may prevent some of the damage free radicals otherwise might cause.

Why is this important to you? Resistance Training increases oxygen intake from 10 to 20 times over the resting state. This greatly increases the generation of free radicals. Antioxidants play the housekeeper's role, "mopping up" free radicals before they get a chance to do harm in your body.

## Super Foods

Mother Nature's perfect foods are the best sources of essential nutrients, antioxidants, major contributors of fiber; fight disease and help you feel satisfied on fewer calories. Even if you were to choose supplements over whole foods, you just cannot make up for the thousands of phytochemicals found in fresh produce. If you concentrate on eating foods that have a lot of nutrients and phytochemicals, you're setting yourself up for a leaner body and healthier life.

1. **FRUITS** - Strawberries, raspberries and blueberries are very high in antioxidants. Blueberries release phytochemicals that speed up the communication between brain cells and help them make dopamine, a key chemical linked to reward and pleasure. Apples are also high in antioxidants and plant nutrients, reducing the risk of some cancers, diabetes, asthma and heart disease.

2. **VEGETABLES -** Broccoli is high on every food expert's list. Along with other cruciferous vegetables, such as kale, Brussels sprouts, cauliflower and cabbage, broccoli contains cancer-fighting compounds called indoles and glycosinolates. Tomatoes are high in lycopene which may help prevent prostate cancer and breast cancer. Dark, leafy green vegetables have a pigment called carotenoids that enhance the body's immune response. The pigment protects skin cells against dangerous ultraviolet rays. These foods are rich in vitamin A and antioxidants. Their anti-inflammatory powers also help block pain.

3. **FISH.** - salmon, mackerel and bluefish (cold water fish) - contain high levels of omega-3 fatty acids. The brain needs these substances to maintain many complex functions. The body requires these specific fatty acids to take care of the heart and protect against stroke.

**FYI:** <u>Benefits Omega-3</u> Helps your body store less fat. In addition, the fat you do store is more readily and easily converted into energy and burned during activity. Increases Size of your cells' fuel-burning furnaces so your metabolic rate rises and you burn more calories every minute of every day. Omega-3's also help your body produce testosterone, the hormone responsible for building new muscle = promotes muscle recovery. If you are not big on fish, consider supplementing these essential nutrients with Prograde's EFA Icon.

4. **WHOLE GRAINS** - There are many whole grains available - couscous, quinoa, bulgur wheat and wheat berries - that provide healthy stores of vitamin B and tons of fiber. (AVOID PROCESSED – enriched –means manufacturers remove the fiber and minerals – just kept the "starch" of the grain, acts similar to sugar when digested – NOT good for fat loss).

**FYI:** Benefits of Fiber

~Keeps you regular - prevents constipation by moving bodily waste through the digestive tract faster, so harmful substances don't have as much contact with the intestinal walls

~Traps carbohydrates to slow their digestion and absorption. Stabilizes blood sugar – keeps insulin levels stable – eliminates cravings and prevents body from going into fat storage mode

~Lowers Cholesterol – reducing risk of heart disease - fiber binds to dietary cholesterol, helping the body to eliminate it. This reduces blood cholesterol levels, which, in turn, reduces cholesterol deposits on arterial walls that

~Reduce risk of obesity - fiber-rich foods are more filling than other foods--so people tend to eat less. Because insoluble fiber is indigestible and passes through the body virtually intact, it provides few calories.

The typical American eats only about 11 grams of fiber a day, you need 25 to 30 grams of fiber a day.

**5. NUTS -** Almonds and walnuts contain powerful anti-inflammatory properties. High in fiber, protein and antioxidants, nuts may reduce the risk of diabetes and may prevent certain cancers. Also, the healthy fats in nuts prevent the accumulation of bad fats in the artery walls. Walnuts and flaxseeds (seeds that have a nutty flavor) contain omega-3 fatty acids, which are good for the heart and brain.

**6. OLIVE OIL -** Extra-virgin olive oil is a wonderful source of good fat (monounsaturated) and powerful plant nutrients. The oil has antioxidant and anti-inflammatory properties and decreases bad forms of cholesterol while boosting good cholesterol.

**7. BEANS AND LENTILS -** High in protein and fiber, beans and lentils contain potent levels of antioxidants. The nutrients in these foods help burn body fat and stabilize blood sugar.

**8. YOGURT** - Yogurt is a rich source of protein, vitamin A, calcium and PROBIOTICS good bacteria that keeps gastrointestinal tract in BALANCE. Since 80% of your body's immune system is located in your intestinal tract, probiotics can be part of your first line of defense against adverse effects of stress, illness and aging Calcium forces fat out of cells and into the bloodstream, where it's more quickly oxidized, or burned off. If your body doesn't get enough calcium, fat cells retain the fat and can grow steadily. Many women don't get enough: Only 14 percent of women ages 20 to 50 get the minimum Recommended Dietary Allowance (RDA) of 1,000 mg of calcium, and only 4 percent of women over 50 meet the 1,200-mg goal.

**9. GREEN TEA -** This beverage is touted for its anti-bacterial and anti-viral effects, and its benefits keep expanding. It's good for the heart and immune system, improves blood flow, is high in antioxidants that fight inflammation, has mood-elevating properties and prevents the absorption of fat. Drink 2 to 3 servings of fresh brewed tea a day.

**10. WATER -** you can survive for 6 weeks without food – you wouldn't last a week without water! **Water helps the body metabolize fat!**
Studies have shown that a decrease in water intake will cause fat deposits to increase, while an increase in water can actually reduce fat deposits.

**Here's why:** The kidneys can't function properly without enough water. When they don't work to capacity, some of their load is dumped onto the liver. One of the livers primary functions is to metabolize (burn) stored fat into usable energy for the body. But, if the liver has to do some of the kidneys. work, it can't operate at full throttle. As a result, it metabolizes less fat, more fat remains stored in the body and weight loss stops.

**Drinking enough water is the best treatment for fluid retention.** When the body gets less water, it perceives this as a threat to survival and begins to hold on to every drop. Water is stored in extra cellular spaces (outside the cells). This shows up as swollen feet, legs, and hands. The best way to overcome water retention is to give the body what it needs – plenty of water. Only than will stored water be released. Excess salt can also be the cause of water retention

**Water helps rid the body of waste.** During weight loss, the body has a lot more waste to get rid of all that metabolized fat must be shed. Again, adequate water helps flush out the waste.

**Water can help relieve constipation.** When the body gets too little water, it siphons what it needs from internal sources. The colon is one primary source. Result? Constipation. But when a person drinks enough water, normal bowel function usually returns.

**How much water is enough?** Average - drink 8 eight-ounce glasses a day (appx. 2 quarts). However, the overweight person needs one additional glass for every 25 pounds of excess weight. Water should preferably be cold. It is absorbed into the system more quickly than warm water. Limit fluid intake after 7pm. Otherwise, you will find yourself going to the bathroom throughout the evening.

## No matter WHAT your GOAL is – Your results are dependent upon how well you are taking care of your body.

Mother Nature's foods are the foundation of a healthy diet.
It is recommend that you consume at least 7 to 10 servings of fruits and veggies a day

### 3 Problems....

Sadly only 10 percent of us are able to follow this advice.

- It difficult to eat this many servings of fruit and vegetables on a consistent basis.
- What if you are a picky eater?
- **Challenge:** How to do this while eating less in order to promote fat loss?

**FACT:** You just don't get enough of the essential vitamins and minerals you need for optimum health through diet alone. You would have to eat 5,000 calories a day, that's about 20 pounds of food!

Because we are most likely not consuming the necessary dosage of nutrients that our bodies need to stay healthy, we need to take some form of nutrient supplement. However, traditional vitamin supplements do not provide us with natural fruit and vegetable extracts, essential fatty acids *or* phytonutrients.

**Prograde's VGF+25 Whole Food Nutrient Complex the simplest way to ensure your nutrient levels are at optimal levels 24 hours a day.**

**The Bottom Line:** Your body cannot burn fat in a malnourish state. A complete Whole Food Nutrient Complex provides your body with the materials necessary to promote a positive, physical change

Get maximum benefits from your nutrition.

Experience the amazing benefits for yourself!

_____

## Complete....

1. List 2 reasons why you need a whole food supplement.

2. Why are antioxidants important to you?

3. List 2 new Super Foods you will begin to incorporate into your menu plan.

# Session Six: Reassessment

**It's time to recognize and celebrate your progress!**

To do this, your body composition and circumference measurements will be assessed. This is just one of several methods to measure what a difference your efforts have made. Take the time to thoughtfully complete this activity. Reflect on the progress you have made and determine where you stand in relation to your initial goals. Make adjustments as needed. Be sure to use the **Solution Discovery Worksheet** in your to assist you in assessing areas of development.

*Reassessment Exercise:* Review your initial Goal Setting Sheet. Review your Personal Commitment Contract.

**List your long-term goals**

Exercise -

Nutrition -

Attitude-

**Be honest** as you ask yourself if you've done well in making progress towards your goal. Have the strategies you laid out to overcome obstacles worked well for you?

What are you doing that works?

Be sure to continue these new habits.

Can you easily overcome these obstacles now with the strategies you've put into place?

If you're still having a tough time tackling your initial short-term goals, it's time to take a look at some of the strategies you've laid out to accomplish these goals. Perhaps these aren't the best strategies for you. Keep this in mind; **if they are not working for you, they are working against you** and it is imperative that they be replaced.

**List the major problem areas/actions that take you further from your goal.**

**What are you doing that you should stop?** Identify at least 2-3 areas of development with a brief strategy to master each one.

1. Exercise obstacle(s):


   Plan of Action:


2. Nutrition obstacle(s):


   Plan of Action:


3. Attitude obstacle(s):

   Plan of Action:



**Remember to continue to take it slowly, pace yourself and expect less than perfection** - Stick with your nutrition and exercise plan even if you experience a slip up. Changing old habits takes consistent effort. You must practice patience as you relearn new behaviors and allow time for your body to positively adjust.

### *Small Behavior Strategies that make a BIG Difference*
Making small changes one at a time is the best strategy. It's not overwhelming and it results in a slower, steadier positive physical change.

- Don't engage in other activities while eating such as watching T.V. driving, reading, or talking on the phone
- Concentrate on the pleasures of the food you eat - the sight, the smell, and the taste. Don't allow eating to be a mindless, unconscious behavior.
- Choose one room for eating, and don't eat while standing or walking around.
- Spend at least 20 minutes eating your meals to allow your brain to trigger a fullness sensation to your stomach. Take small bites, chew your food completely, set fork down between bites.
- Don't always leave a clean plate. Pay more attention to your hunger. It's OK to leave something if you feel satisfied before you're finished. Put it away for tomorrow if you want.
- If you can't eat "just one" of certain foods, don't buy that food. Never eat out of a bag or box. Take out a measured/counted quantity of food and put it in a bowl. This way, you know exactly how much you're having.
- Try at least one new food every week. If you're bored with what you're eating, you're more likely to give up
- Don't go grocery shopping on an empty stomach. Shop from a prepared list.
- Buy foods that require preparation. Ready-to-eat foods have little to no nutritional value.
- Incorporate small bouts of exercise into your daily routine. Aim for 30 minutes a day. Try taking the stairs, parking further away, walking to the grocery store, hand-washing your car, playing an sport with your children, or simply go for a 10 minute walk three times a day.
- Make exercise a **priority**, not an inconvenience.

**It is very important to recognize and reward yourself for the progress that you have made.** List some non-food rewards:

I have accomplished:

This is my reward:

I accomplished:

This is my reward:

**Create a goal short term goal for the next week:**

When I accomplish:

This is my reward:

Remember your transformation is a journey, not a destination. Accomplishing any goal requires a lifelong commitment. Expect to set new goals and discover new areas of improvement. The reality is, most goals do change over time. Goals should be changed in response to things that happen in or around you. Your goals are a direct reflection of where you are and where you're going in life. Change is just part of the process. The key is to break your goals down into simple steps that you can complete. This allows you to make measurable progress and established a forward momentum.

### Don't forget to Reward Yourself

When you were a kid, and you did something well, every now and then you got a reward. Motivating, right? Reaching your fitness goals is no different. Use that same logic to make your weight-loss journey more pleasant — and your goal more attainable. Set mini-goals, then reward yourself when you meet them. When you reward yourself for your efforts – not the outcome – on a regular basis, you will continue to motivate yourself to stick with your program.

If you don't celebrate small, everyday lifestyle changes, there will be times when your fitness goal seems so far away that you'll become frustrated or be tempted to give up. Having little stops to celebrate along the way makes that journey more pleasant — and your goal more likely to be achieved. When you meet one of your mini-milestones, be sure to give yourself a reward.

**For under $5, why not …**

- Sip on a cup of an exotic herbal tea in the sun.
- Finish the day with a long, candlelit soak in the tub.
- Enjoy a leisurely Sunday morning — turn your phone off and spend the morning in your pajamas reading a book or devouring a few magazines.
- Savor a celebratory glass of wine with dinner.
- Rent your favorite movie

**For under $10, why not …**

- Open a "pamper me" bank account: Deposit $10 for every week you've stuck to your nutrition and exercise plan, or for every pound of fat you've lost. Save up for a day at the spa.
- Splurge on a bouquet of flowers just for you.
- Take the time to give yourself a full manicure, complete with a new shade of nail polish.
- Buy a relaxation tape and use it daily.
- Take a trip to the book store and buy a book you are eager to read.

**For $20 to $45, why not …**

- Pay your neighbor's teenager to do your grocery shopping for you. Just make a list, relax.
- String a hammock up in the backyard and spend an afternoon napping in the sun.
- Call your distant friends.
- Enjoy a new haircut or color.
- Get a makeover.

**For over $50, why not …**

- Devote the entire day to a shopping spree for a new pair of shoes.
- Splurge on a bottle of new perfume — just because you deserve it.
- Rent a sailboat with friends and spend the day soaking up ocean breezes.
- Sign up for a membership to your favorite art gallery, or subscribe to a theater company for the next season.
- Hire a maid for the day — to cook and clean while you kick back.
- Take that vacation you've been putting off.
- Get a massage.
- You are looking great – have your picture taken by a professional.
- Invest in a Personal Trainer - take the extra step to ensure you achieve a tone, sculpted body.

# Secrets to Accelerate Goal Achievement

1. Commitment – How important is this to you?
2. Enthusiasm and passion – What's your REASON for doing this?
3. Thinking about your goal A LOT – at the very least, on a daily basis.
4. Regularly working with and getting help from positive sources of support – talk to or read about those who have been successful
5. Moving out of your comfort zone
6. Letting go of old ways of doing things
7. Taking lots and lots of action – every day you are moving, are you moving closer to or further from your goal?
8. Correct as you go – LEARN from each experience. If one thing doesn't work, try something else.

## Recognize Your Efforts

When you are moving with great momentum towards achieving your goals, it is important to appreciate yourself for the big and small changes you're making. There may be times when you feel like you're falling short of your daily plan or even going backwards. You may even find yourself criticizing your progress. This the best time for self-appreciation, especially if you've had a tough day with some setbacks. You need to realize and anticipate that there will be good days, OK days and plain old bad days! Begin recognizing and appreciating yourself for your commitment, your drive, your focus and patience.

# Session Seven: Food Label

You're grocery shopping ---and you're bombarded with choices. Which type of cheese has the least amount of fat? Which type of cereal is a good source of fiber? What's the difference between skim and whole milk? Which fruit has more vitamin C—canned applesauce or peaches? You'll find the answers on the Nutrition Facts Food Label. Labels tell a lot about food. They don't suggest what foods to eat—that's your decision. But labels can help you make your "personal best" food choices—choices that benefit you as you pursue your fitness goals.

Discover how any food - including your favorites - can fit into a healthful diet in sensible amounts. Maximize your trips to the grocery store by using labels to make healthy food choices.

**Start with the Serving Size**
The first place to start when you examine the food or nutrition label is the serving size and the number of servings in the package. Serving sizes are standardized to make it easier to compare similar foods; they are provided in familiar units, such as cups or pieces. The size of the serving on the food package influences the number of calories and all the nutrient amounts listed on the top part of the label. Pay attention to the serving size, especially how many servings there are in the food package. Then ask yourself, "How many servings am I consuming"? In the sample label, one serving equals one cup. If you ate the whole package, you would eat two cups. That doubles the calories and other nutrient numbers, including the %Daily Values as shown in the sample label.

## Check the Calories

The calorie section of the label can help you manage your weight (gain, lose or maintain.) The number of servings you consume determines the number of calories you actually eat. In the sample label, there are 250 calories in one serving. How many calories from fat are there in ONE serving? What if you ate the whole package?

## Limit These Nutrients

The nutrients listed first are the ones we generally eat in adequate amounts, or even too much. Eating too much **saturated fat, trans fat, cholesterol**, or **sodium** may increase your risk of certain chronic diseases, like heart disease, some cancers, or high blood pressure. Important: Keep your intake of these nutrients as low as possible. Limit sodium to no more than 2400 mg a day, cholesterol to 300 mg and avoid foods that have more than 2 grams of saturated fat.

## Carbohydrates

Carbohydrates include sugars, complex carbohydrates, and fiber. A quality carbohydrate should also have fiber and sugar. Try to avoid carbohydrates with zero fiber. A quality carbohydrate has at least 1/6 as fiber – For example; 20 grams of carbohydrate would have around 3 - 4 grams of fiber.

## Sugars

Sugars include naturally occurring sugars such as fructose in fruit and lactose in dairy products as well as added sugars such as sucrose (table sugar). Nutritionally they are just simple carbohydrates that are just contributing empty calories.

## Proteins

Most Americans get more protein than they need. Where there is animal protein, there is also fat and cholesterol. Eat small servings of lean meat, fish and poultry. Use skim or low-fat milk, yogurt and cheese. Try vegetable proteins like beans, grains and cereals.

## Nutrients to Increase

Most Americans don't get enough dietary **fiber, vitamin A, vitamin C, calcium**, and **iron** in their diets. Eating enough of these nutrients can improve your health and help reduce the risk of some diseases and conditions. For example, getting enough calcium may reduce the risk of osteoporosis. Eating a diet high in dietary fiber promotes healthy bowel function and promotes weight loss. Additionally, a diet rich in fruits, vegetables, and grain products that contain dietary fiber, may reduce the risk of heart disease. Aim for 20 to 35 grams of fiber a day.

## Footnotes

This part tells you the amount you should get of each nutrient if you take in 2,000 or 2,500 calories in one day. When the full footnote does appear, it will always be the same. It doesn't change from product to product, because it shows recommended dietary advice for all Americans--it is not about a specific food product.

## Daily Values

The % Daily Values (%DVs) are based on the Daily Value recommendations for key nutrients but only for a 2,000 calorie daily diet. Use the %DV as a frame of reference based around the calories you consume, even if they are more or less than 2,000 calories. Anything that is 5%DV or less is low for all nutrients, you want to limit these (fat, saturated fat, cholesterol, and sodium), and for those that you want to consume in greater amounts (fiber, calcium, potassium etc.) the label shows, 20%DV or more is high for all nutrients.

**Example:** Look at the amount of Total Fat in one serving listed on the sample label. Is 18%DV contributing a lot or a little to your fat limit of 100% DV? It is 18%DV, which is below 20%DV, not yet high, but what if you ate the whole package (two servings)? You would double that amount, eating 36% of your daily allowance for Total Fat. Coming from just one food, that amount leaves you with 64% of your fat allowance (100%-36%=64%) for all of the other foods you eat that day, snacks and drinks included.

**Finally, Check the Ingredients List**
Ingredients are listed in descending order of predominance. This means that the first ingredient is the most prevalent in the product, while the last ingredient has the least amount in the product. The ingredient list can help you identify 'hidden' ingredients, like added sugars, trans-fats (hydrogenated oils) and coconut oil or palm oil, which are high in saturated fat.

## Ingredient List *Red Flags*:

- Enriched anything. Enriched means the food was stripped of vital nutrients.
- A protein where the fat calories are half of or more than the total calories (unless, of course, you are looking at a bottle of olive oil)
- A carbohydrate where sugars are half or more of the total grams of carbohydrates (ex. Carbohydrates 12g, sugars 6g.)
- Avoid partially hydrogenated oils (also known as trans-fatty acids) and hydrogenated oils (as opposed to partially hydrogenated).

## Complete while comparing at least 2 food labels from home

1. What information do you look at first? Why?

2. Which item has the most calories per serving?

3. Which item has the largest amount of fiber?

4. Which item has the least percentage of total fat?

5. Which item has the largest percentage of sodium?

6. Which item has an abundance of vitamins?

7. How will reading labels help you to eat more supportively?

# Session Eight: Healthy Fast Food

Americans are spending HALF of their food dollars on meals purchased outside of the home. This fact makes the art of making healthy fast food choices a necessary survival skill in order for you to stay within your calorie guidelines and five percent of your recommended percentages of protein, carbohydrate and fat. With the popularity of fast food and the number of new restaurants on the rise, there are more food choices than ever. But you still need information about food other than what is on the menu.

The term "*Fast Food*" is commonly associated with hamburgers, greasy french fries, and cola. However, popular family restaurant menu items can be ordered "*to go*" without waiting for their preparation or standing in a long line. You can even pay with a credit card over the phone if you're in a real hurry. Overall, fast food does not have to be high-calorie and high-fat food.

**May I take your order, please?**
What you order is the key. It's very easy to eat an entire day's worth of fat, salt, and calories in just one fast food meal. But it's also possible to make wise choices and eat a fairly healthy meal.

Tips to help you choose well

- Know that an average fast-food meal can run as high as 1800 calories or more

- Know the nutritional value of the foods you order. Sometimes "good choices", are higher in the nutrients or calories. Fat-free or Low-Fat items may have plenty of sugar or salt.

- If you're having fast-food for one meal, make all the other meals that day contain the right portion of lean protein, starchy carb and fibrous carb.

- Know your food is cooked. Chicken and fish can be good choices - but not if they are breaded and deep fried.

- Avoid jumbo, giant, deluxe, biggie-sized or super-sized. Larger portions mean more calories, fat, cholesterol, sugar and salt.

## When Dining Out

Tempting menus, extra large portions and festive atmospheres make it easy to overlook supportive eating. Splurging once in awhile is okay, but you'll begin to pack on pounds if you make it a habit. It is possible to enjoy yourself and still make supportive choices. Following a few simple rules when eating out can make it possible to maintain your nutrition plan.

1. **Order food to go** – Studies show that people tend to consume more food when they are not eating at their own kitchen tables. Take home and have the option of providing a healthier side dish such as fruit or vegetables.
2. **KNOW** where you will go and what you will eat ahead of time
3. **EAT before you GO**

4. **Avoid buffets** – They are invitations to OVEREATING
5. **CHOOSE Wisely** - use the guidelines of Supportive Menu Design
6. **Avoid the BREAD Basket**
7. **ASK how food is prepared** – ask for baked, broiled, roasted, poached or steamed
8. **Don't be afraid to special order** – Ask for your vegetables and main dishes to be served without the sauces.
9. **Watch portion size** – Servings can be 3-5 times more than what you need.
10. **Share** –Sample what you want while avoiding the temptation to overindulge.
11. **WATER** - Drink at least one full-glass of water before eating. You'll feel full sooner, you will eat less.
12. **Order an appetizer** and a salad as your meal.
13. **Front Load** your meal with a nutritious salad or bowl of soup to take the edge off your appetite
14. **Order sauce and dressing on the side** –Control calories and enjoy the taste
15. **Order first**. You're less likely to be influenced by the choices of your companions
16. **Take the time to enjoy your meal**. Savor the flavors and textures of your food, and enjoy the company you're with. When you eat slowly, you give your body's internal clock the time it needs to know when you've had enough. When you're full, stop eating.
17. *Save dessert for later* – A great trick to play is instead of ordering dessert at a restaurant, go somewhere else. By the time you get there, you will not be as hungry and will end up eating half or even skipping dessert entirely.

You can dine out on occasion while remaining true to your goals. The key is to plan ahead, choose wisely and you'll find foods that fit into your meal plan.

### Slip-ups

Sometimes we slip up. We overeat or pick less healthy foods because they sound good, we're stressed, or we just feel like it. Supportive eating is a lifelong goal. If one meal isn't healthy, make sure the next one is. If you overdo it one day, put 100% effort into the following day. And don't forget to work in exercise to make up for those extra calories.

REMEMBER: Supportive Nutrition is not all or nothing; it's about balance and moderation. "It isn't one food, one day, that will make you fat. Just remember, it all adds up."

## Complete….

1. How often do you eat Fast Food? How much do you spend per day/week/month? (I don't know is not an answer.)

2. What modifications do you make or can you make to your order?

3. What do you typically order?

4. Use the following links to find out the nutrition values of the meals you eat out. Be sure to record total calories, fat, sugar and sodium for each item/meal. Also take note of ingredients when listed.

**BURGER KING** http://www.burgerking.com/Food/Nutrition/downloads/nutritionals.pdf The Whopper JR or Hamburger both have 310 calories and 13 grams of fat. The Chicken Whopper has 410 calories and 7 grams of fat. Avoid the Ranch and Zesty Onion dip at all cost...15 grams of fat per serving.

**Chick-Fil-A** http://www.chick-fil-a.com/MenuTable.asp?Category=specialties Chick-fil-a makes it easy to understand what is in each food item. Their nutrition facts can be read as if you are looking at a food label...look at the % RDA. A plus for chick-fil-a, you can now swap out the fries for fresh fruit--yeah somebody gets it!

**HARDEES** www.hardees.com/lowcarb.pdf Beware of Hardees new low carb items, although low in carbs, the fat content in the low carb thickburger(lettuce burger), the low carb chicken club have a n amazing 24-50 grams of fat. www.hardees.com/nutrition/

**KFC** http://www.yum.com/nutrition/menu.asp?brandID_Abbr=2_KFC Get the skinny on Kentucky Fried Chicken's Menu items. One of there better looking meals is the Oven Roasted Strips Meal: 3 Oven Roasted Strips, Green Beans, Seasoned Rice. Only 7 grams of total fat, but be careful this meal is loaded with 100% of your daily recommended intake of Sodium.

**McDonalds** http://www.mcdonalds.com/app_controller.nutrition.categories.nutrition.index.html

**Starbucks** http://www.starbucks.com/retail/nutrition_info.asp Beware of any beverage that contains the words crème' or whip those words equate to high fat and 100-200 more calories per 16oz drink. Topping that list is the Strawberries and Crème' Frap Grande(16oz) with whip at 580 calories and 17g of fat or the White Hot Chocolate with whip at 580 calories and 28g of fat.

**Taco Bell** www.tacobell.com/nutrition.htm Total fat calories for two regular beef tacos with a regular side of nachos and cheese is a whopping 39 grams of fat. Your daily recommended is typically 68 grams or less.

**WENDY's** www.wendys.com/food/index.jsp?country=US&lang=EN Think twice about ordering the Homestyle Chicken Strip Salad, it has 22 grams of fat without the dressing, add 1 packet of ranch dressing and pack a total of 45 grams of fat into one sitting.

**PANERA BREAD** http://panerabread.com/menu/ OR http://panerabread.com/pdf/nutr-guide.pdf Panera Bread's delicious sandwiches range between 590 – 1100 calories...saturated fat is between 11 and 56 grams......this not including your choice of side.

# Session 9 Master your Motivation

## If the "why" is big enough then we can always find the "how."

Motivation is a powerful tool for success. The degree to which you can remain motivated and continue to make forward progress determines whether you realize the goals that you establish. But the reward for being motivated isn't just raw goal accomplishment. The following benefits of being motivated are numerous - and they can change your life.

**Creativity:** Motivated people think more clearly. They focus more intellectual resources on their current project, and the result is more creativity.

**Energy:** People who are motivated actually need less sleep - not because they're on a constant adrenaline rush but because they possess a genuine, energizing excitement.

**Flexibility:** Motivated folks have discovered that flexibility is a developed skill that doesn't depend on circumstances. When their circumstances change, they're more open to bending to deal with the situation rather than being rigid about an outcome.

**Health:** People who have a positive feeling about their life and its potential have reason to get and stay healthy. They have experienced the difference in energy and healthfulness during non-motivated times, and they prefer the motivated lifestyle.

**Magnetism:** A motivated lifestyle is attractive, and motivated people have a certain magnetism. Others are naturally drawn to winners who are energizing by nature and habit.

**Momentum:** Motivation is self-perpetuating. It gathers speed as it rolls along. Living out your motivation gets easier because it becomes a habit.

**Multiplication**: Motivation is contagious - it spreads and multiplies. The people around the one who is motivated "catch" that motivation.

**Recognition:** When people live out a motivated lifestyle, they stand out. Others respect them for their achievements, admire their spunk, and, because they want to be associated with winners, offer their assistance.

**Optimism:** Motivated individuals have found out that optimism opens more doors than negativity. They have discovered a life pattern of finding the silver lining or the potential in any turn of events. They aren't thrown off course by change. They find the good in everything.

**Productivity:** Motivated people get more done. They move with a spring in their step, and they attack tasks with enthusiasm. They move quickly, deliberately, and with a concern for maintaining a can-do attitude along the way.

**Stability:** Folks with motivation are focused and are not easily distracted or dissuaded from their destinations. They are tuned in to the object of their motivation.

# Incentive: The Mother of Motivation

The fact is, however, that motivation just doesn't last very long. Motivation tends to be kind of an exterior thing. Inspiration, on the other hand, is more INTERNAL—it has more staying power. It needs stimulation from time to time, but it's something we draw forth from WITHIN rather than pasted on the outside.

It is our mission is "to inform, **inspire** and empower people to be the very best version of their self—physically and personally. Everything we do is with this mission in mind. In class, we share new ideas and sometimes we remind you of things you already know. We do our best to keep the fire of inspiration burning by keeping what you know and what you care about in the forefront of your mind.

We don't try to motivate you as much as we strive to inspire you and help you draw forth your own inspiration—inspiration that leads to action.

Motivation -- and passion -- begins and ends with incentive. You have to know what you want and why you want it, and achieving it may be reward in and of itself. This is called "intrinsic" reward. "Extrinsic" rewards are such things as money, prizes or numbers on a scale. In both cases, the rewards serve as incentive to continue.

Recognize incentive as a powerful motivating force. What is your reason, your incentive?

If you find yourself lacking motivation, it may be that your incentive lacks passion or emotion. If you decide to create powerful, passion filled goals, you will probably need to make changes in yourself in order to achieve them.

How has it changed as you have progressed through this course? (Review initial Goal Sheet)

How can you add more passion or emotion to this incentive to prevent your motivation from waning?

# Session 10 Plateau Busters

## Everything works, but nothing works forever

Hitting a plateau is a common experience. It can be one of the most de-motivating things to happen. Plateaus are the number one reason why people abandon exercise. They bring on feelings of discouragement, confusion, and utter frustration. Thankfully, overcoming it is easy... all you need to do is prepare for it to happen and know the steps to take to overcome it.

### What is a plateau?

The human body has a regulatory mechanism that works to keep the amount of energy you consume in balance with the amount of energy you use. In other words, the body does not like to lose weight! the slowing or halt of fat/weight loss **in spite of** exercise consistency and consistent, proper food intake.

Look at the experience of a plateau, as a ***good thing!*** Your body telling you "I am ready for the next stage"- "I have conquered this current routine" – *"**Give me something new!!**"* This is when fitness gets fun and you can add creativity to your routine.

The human body is amazingly adaptable for a variety of reasons. What you first need to do is identify the reason for the adaptation and make then proceed with the proper changes.

## *Plateaus: The Reasons & The Solutions*

### Lowering calories too far...

"It takes calories to burn calories," which is true both internally and externally. Internally, the body simply slows its metabolic rate (burns fewer calories) when it senses a decrease in food intake. The body still functions correctly, but requires fewer calories, creating hunger and preventing fat loss. Externally, the body is tricked into doing less,(i.e., you get lazy, tired and therefore, move less and more economically).

### What to do...

To prevent a plateau, keep your calories *slightly* below the amount recommended for maintenance to keep your metabolism and energy levels high during exercise and daily activities. A deficit greater than 500 to 700 calories makes it much more difficult to maintain lean muscle.

### Loss of lean body mass

Lean body mass uses up to eight times the calories as fat does. Therefore, loss of enough of this fat burning commodity (muscle) dramatically lowers metabolism and brings fat loss to a screeching halt.

### What to do...

Keep your body nourished with supportive foods and a quality multivitamin. Follow your exercise recommendations; resistance training at least 3 times a week, no more than 20-30 minutes of cardio.

### Net weight loss

The less you weigh the fewer calories it takes to move your body, even during exercise.

### What to do...

Concentrate on increasing lean muscle through resistance training. This is an ideal way to compensate for the fat loss of calories, due to net weight loss, and enhance your look.

### Body becomes Efficient

The body is required to make hundreds of internal changes to adjust to different workloads. Each of these reactions consumes calories. Therefore, once the body stops repairing muscle from exercise or adding new cellular machinery, the calories burned to make these changes are no longer spent and the amount of energy your body uses decreases.

### What to do...

Never let your body get used to exercise. Keep it guessing by changing frequency, intensity, type or time of exercise. When training for

## Overtraining

More exercise is not always better. Just as in under-eating, overtraining may decrease the amount of calories you burn. This is partially due to adaptive thermogenesis, (a survival mechanism). In other words, there may be a point of diminishing returns, when an increase in exercise energy expenditure is negated by an equal decrease in non-exercise energy expenditure. This negates the additional work, at least until expenditure is dramatically increased and/or calories decreased.

### What to do...

Take at least seven days off from your regular exercise routine (this should be done every 12 weeks, regardless). Start back with less and a different type of work and increase only as necessary (e.g., the least amount of specific work to initiate change). Your metabolism and daily activities will reset and increase again.

## Enhanced physical condition

When you are in overall better shape, your system is more efficient - burns fewer calories to operate. The primary benefit of exercise is to improve health through an appropriate regime. Improved health can cause a slower resting metabolic rate. In other words, fewer calories are burned during normal daily activities. This is partially due to an increase in cardiopulmonary efficiency (e.g., lower resting heart rate).

### What to do...

Stick with your goal of staying healthy. Concentrate on exercise intensity and type changes for a longer "after-burn" (calories burned above the normal resting metabolic rate after exercise).

Just as a well-tuned car gets better fuel economy, a well-tuned body can also thrive on less fuel (calories) when consistently challenged. By making a few changes, you can jumpstart your routine and see positive results in no time.

Remember, the best ways to stave off a weight loss plateau involve boosting your metabolism, not decreasing your calories. Consider the following **Plateau Busters**:

- Reassess exercise time and intensity. If you've walked 30 minutes, three times a week for a few weeks, that's great! But it's time to add small bouts of extra intensity so 20 minutes now feels challenging. Do the extra rep or two, increase your range of motion, and increase resistance as you get stronger.
- Reassess exercise activities. Try new activities to cause muscles to be challenged and burn more calories.
- Consistency. Improvement and change occur when you do things often. Stopping and starting all the time will kill any momentum you need to succeed. You must find ways to stay in the game. Moderate forms of exercise, done consistently, provide far better results than the occasional full-body pummeling. A lifestyle that includes multiple forms of exercise five to six days a week guarantees results.
- Avoid the scale. Focus on inches lost and the leaner you are becoming. Your body fat percentage will decrease significantly *over time*.
- Make sure you are eating smaller, more frequent meals. Every time you eat the right amount and type of foods, you give your metabolism a small boost.
- Reassess the short-term goals that you made in Session Two to be sure you've selected the right strategies. Perhaps you need to re-evaluate the goals you made and come up with new solutions.
- Use your Fitness Journal to track and view how far you've come and how well you've done. This positive feedback will hold you accountable and help you stay motivated.

# Complete....

1    What is a Plateau?

2   List two reasons why a Plateau occurs?


3   What can you do to avoid a plateau?


# Session 11: Overcoming Unwanted Behaviors

You decide you want to improve your body and live a healthier lifestyle. You map out a nutritional strategy, design your own workout schedule and you embark on the journey to a leaner, more toned physique…and it starts working! But the minute you begin getting results, you fall off the wagon. You binge, you skip workouts, you cheat. What's most perplexing (and upsetting) is that you know what you should do… but no matter how hard you try, you can't get yourself to do it! It's as if some unseen force is sabotaging you and controlling your behavior like you were a puppet on a string.

You are actually *blocking* your own success with feelings of being overwhelmed as you get closer to your goal. You allow yourself to become dominated by these unproductive feelings and your state of mind affects your actions. You're not able to accept the feelings of joy and power associated with your accomplishments. Denying feelings of accomplishment and success, results in producing highly ineffective and self-sabotaging behaviors. The behaviors are self-sabotaging because you're responding opposite to what is required to reach your goals. Fear of success occurs because negative self-talk and negative messages from others still dominate your beliefs and attitude. What is your chance of success or advancement if you allow others to affect your thoughts and behavior?

Realize that your effort in eliminating negative self-talk and negative beliefs from others is aimed at <u>improving your self-confidence</u>. Developing your inner resources, your self-esteem and self-respect, will motivate you to accept feelings of success on a continual basis.

> ~ Bravely overcoming discouraging feelings about yourself by eliminating self-defeating words from your vocabulary is one way to overcome fear of success.
> ~ Another way is to disregard self-defeating statements from others.
> ~ Success is achieved by continually expressing positive self-talk directed toward developing your enthusiasm, self-esteem, and vitality. "I can do it," "Great job," and "Well done" are expressions of your vitality, influencing the course of your life.

Changing your way of thinking about success activates your courage to solve problems and achieve goals. Instead of letting your problems get the better of you, take control and energize your courage by saying, "I am determined to reach my goals," and "My self-confidence and self-respect are so strong that I will move forward in life." These courageous affirmations will enable you to master and take control of your emotional, mental, and physical qualities to create passion in your life.

Your commitment to eliminate fear of success, and change your thoughts and actions, is a personal choice. Although internal, negative self-talk and discouraging words from others seem to surround you, focus your thoughts and actions in positive, productive ways.

When you experience rough times, discouraging words from others or negative self-talk, don't let yourself get down. Face the challenge and keep moving forward. Believe in yourself and use encouraging self-talk to help you become enthusiastic about changing your behavior and attitude.

| **3 ways to overcome fear of success:** |
| --- |
| 1. Continually tell yourself that you welcome challenges. Stand ready and willing to challenge yourself to your maximum capacity. Move forward in your communication |

by *deleting* all negative self-talk.

2.  Believe that whatever you set out to accomplish, you will give it 100%. Stop providing excuses to blame yourself, becoming disempowered from achieving your goals and increasing your self-esteem. Believe that your "pride of accomplishment" motivates you to eliminate all the "should's," "ought's," and "must's," from your vocabulary.

3.  Be the best you can. Continually "see" yourself in an evolving way. Stretch every mental, emotional, and physical fiber within you. Believe and feel that you are one dynamite, ecstatic, and powerful person. Remember, your beliefs impact the way you feel and act.

When we consider actually moving toward our heart's desire, a part of us automatically looks ahead to the possible consequences - especially the negative ones. Our "comfort zone" glooms onto these negative consequences. The comfort zone argues it's the actions that will bring on the negative consequences.

You have the *choice to* control negativity and self-sabotaging behavior by creating positive beliefs and envisioning positive outcomes. Try a strategy called "thought stopping". You can use this to change the direction when you find yourself slipping into a negative thought pattern. Say to yourself, with a loud and firm inner voice: STOP! Once you've done this, it's important to replace your previous thought with a more positive statement and image. Clearly acknowledge which statements cause you to feel pain or threat, and which statements allow you to feel success, joy and happiness.

When people unnecessarily stress themselves by thinking that they have no control over a controllable situation, they need to use their inner voice to shout out the word "STOP." Then, change track and think about how the situation can be redirected.

When you attach specific positive words to positive feelings and experiences, you can recall positive feelings at will by using those words. Try to apply a positive affirmation for yourself. Use a positive statement; attach it to feelings of success, joy, and happiness by making the effort to FEEL these emotions. For example, "When I challenge and encourage myself, I consistently move toward my goals with a success attitude, 'I Can I Will.' "

Recite the statement to yourself several times. Each time, experience the positive feelings the statement generates. When you anchor positive words or statements to positive feelings, you can recall the positive feeling anytime you desire and create more positive outcomes, consistently.

Challenge yourself. Stop your self-sabotaging thoughts and behaviors. Practicing thought stopping on a continual basis allows you to eliminate negative thoughts to become more aware of your feelings of accomplishment, self-acceptance, and of positive choice and change. Your new, bright thoughts and feelings of pleasure, joy and happiness drive you toward your destination of success. Positive feelings and beliefs increase your self-worth and self-esteem, empowering you to take action.

## Simple Steps, Big Results

1.  Don't sabotage your best efforts to be fit with negative self talk/behaviors

2. Take responsibility for your thoughts, health and life
3. Focus on simple, daily steps to reach your goals

These three strategies are the solution to every self-sabotaging habit that interferes with your goals to look and feel your very best. We are often our own worst enemies, declaring that we want to lose weight, eat better, or have more energy, and all the while continuing to eat foods that work against our efforts, manufacturing excuses for why we don't have time to exercise, or blame others for our eating habits, all of which divert us from reaching our goals.

What you need to realize is that healthy and fit living doesn't take a total life overhaul. It requires a change in your priorities. We are all living reflections of our priorities. Very simply, when health is a priority, we eat well and exercise. We will adopt lifelong healthy eating habits if losing weight and maintaining the loss means enough to us.

You have progressed through a course that has guided you thus far. Therefore it is safe to say that you want good health or a more trim and fit body to be your priority. But the big question is…Have you MADE it priority?

No matter what you say is important to you, it's where you direct your attention, spend your time and put your effort that speaks the loudest about what is most essential to you in your life.

## Complete….
Identify the "self-sabotaging" fear of success in your life

1. What do I think will happen if I achieve the results I desrie?

2. What would successful results look like?

3. In what ways do I feel undeserving of successful results?

4. Who am I afraid of hurting or intimidating if I achieve success?

5.  What do I think is lacking to keep me from sustaining successful results?

6.  Have I ever put myself down for achieving success in this area?

After looking at the negative consequences of the fear of success, **identify the beliefs** that lead you to this fear. Next, **refute** them if they are irrational, and **replace** them with rational beliefs. If your beliefs are negative self-talk, replace them with positive self-talk.

# Session 12: New Beginnings

*WOW! You are truly amazing! Look how far you've come!*
## You have achieved extraordinary success!

Know that the process of self improvement does not end here! This is merely a time to review and find some new areas where you can focus your attention and continue to achieve.

### Reassessment Exercise:

Achieving your Short-Term Goal: Review your Goal Setting sheet, Session 6 Reassessment and Weekly Reflection activities. How well have you done in tackling your goal. How have the new and revised strategies you laid out to overcome these obstacles, worked for you? Have you mastered the initial areas of development? If your answer is yes, it's time to move on and create some new goals.

If your answer is no, read on....If you're still having a tough time tackling your initial short-term goals, it's time again to take a look at the strategies you've laid out to accomplish these goals. Once again, you can use the **Solution Discovery Worksheet** in your <u>Fitness Toolbox</u> to assist you in assessing areas of development.

**Be honest** as you ask yourself if you've done well in making progress towards your goal. Have the strategies you laid out to overcome obstacles worked well for you?

What are you doing that works?

**What is NOT working? What strategies are working against you?**

**What are you doing that you should stop?** Identify at least 2-3 areas of development with a brief strategy to master each one.

1. Exercise obstacle(s):


   Plan of Action:


2. Nutrition obstacle(s):


   Plan of Action:


3. Attitude obstacle(s):

   Plan of Action:

**Choose 2-3 NEW areas of development to begin focusing on**

1. Exercise problem(s):

Short-term goals:

2. Nutrition problem(s):

Short-term goals:

3. Attitude problem(s):

Short-term goals:

### The Basic Plan: Persistence

All successful weight controllers persist. They exercise despite the usual excuses of time, effort money and aches and pains. They persist even though they live in the age of fast food and….they persist after a vacation full of deviations or a holiday full of unresisted temptations.

### The Choice of Acceptance

Have you reached this stage? In the acceptance stage, people settle in for the long haul. They experience a peaceful sense of resolve about the composition of their body. They feel comfortable and have a clear direction for handling their challenging biology's. They also refine their knowledge of nutrition in this stage. Their understanding of factors that affect fat loss and metabolism becomes clear as well. They recognize and even expect that their will at times struggle with their ability to focus or stay committed. This most likely happens when they go on vacations or when their schedules are disrupted by illness or travel. You will know you are in this stage when you can view exercise as either enjoyable or at least acceptable. You exercise on a consistent basis. You consistently monitor your intake of supportive foods. You actually prefer to eat supportively and you are willing to exert yourself effectively in restaurants and other social situations to ensure that your food works for you. You are unwilling to put yourself in a position where you would be mindless again about your eating, exercise and body composition. You have made a very active choice to pursue the life of a lean, fit, healthy person.

What is your plan to continue your progress or to maintain your new body?

What would you do if you found yourself 8 pounds heavier than usual?

Maintaining lost weight can often be exciting and challenging. It is important look at lifestyle changes as permanent, not temporary actions. You must continue to apply these healthy habits even after you lose the body fat.

Focus on the importance of continuing with the same principles you've learned and lived in the past 11 sessions -- for life. You've acquired time-tested strategies people have successfully used to lose weight *permanently*. You've also learned effective tactics for coping with weight loss plateaus and those times when you have difficulty meeting your goals.

**Tips to help you stay motivated on your journey towards permanent weight loss.**

- ➤ Practice continuous self-monitoring with your Fitness Journal.
- ➤ Make regular and frequent contacts with an outside source of support.
- ➤ Include daily physical activity (resistance training and cardio) for at least 30-45 minutes, three to five days a week.
- ➤ Make regular exercise a PRIORITY, a scheduled appointment, NOT an option.
- ➤ Stay focused on improving health and energy, with fat loss being a nice accompaniment.
- ➤ Set small daily/weekly goals
- ➤ Replace fatty and sugary foods with more healthy substitutions like fruits, vegetables, whole-grains, and other high-fiber foods.
- ➤ Frequently monitor portion sizes and hunger -- this is important in today's world of "super-size" restaurant portions.
- ➤ Find ways to make fitness fun. For example, join a walking or hiking group, a soccer league, or take dance classes. Don't fear trying new activities.
- ➤ Eat at least 4-6 meals a day and do not skip meals.
- ➤ Use Solution Discovery strategies when old behaviors return to haunt you. Make an effort to succeed at creating and re-assessing goals.
- ➤ Recognize that it is a continuous, life-long journey to pursue better health, not a temporary "diet".
- ➤ Never give up! Do not allow occasional slip-ups to end your progress.
- ➤ Accept that the time-tested principles of weight loss, while not always exciting, are the only ones that work permanently.
- ➤ Separate your body size from your self-worth. Recognize that your value is about a lot more than a number. When your attitude shifts to self-acceptance at any size, weight loss and maintaining it becomes more natural, and much easier.
- ➤ Develop passions, interests, and hobbies to help you focus on things other than food.
- ➤ Find and develop creative ways to manage stress effectively.
- ➤ Ban the words "never" and "always" from your health vocabulary. That is, everything in moderation. It's not realistic to say you'll never eat ice cream again or that you will always exercise every day. In short, you must give up perfection, but remain focused without it.
- ➤ Reflect daily. Learn and relearn these tools and strategies and continually reinforce them. It takes many years to learn behaviors that lead to weight gain, yet it usually takes only a short time to lose weight. Therefore, you can expect that from time to time, destructive eating patterns will resurface. Seeking outside sources of support, developing interests, forgiving yourself, and reassessing goals greatly helps to conquer these times.

The overwhelming majority of successful weight maintainers don't report highly restrictive diets and fad diets as factors they used to achieve permanent weight loss. Despite the fact that dietary change is the most commonly reported method to lose weight, the greatest predictors of permanent weight loss have more to do with regular exercise, changing behaviors, positive mindset, continuous self-assessment, and seeking outside support.

The take home message is that the majority of successful weight maintainers have been highly creative and persistent about finding and applying what works for them. You must learn constantly about what works for you and develop your own personal tricks and put them into action.

Commitment is the ultimate decider of permanent physical change. It takes commitment to stick to your new, healthy lifestyle. When you are committed, you will do anything to reach your goal, no matter how hard, tedious, boring, scary...you will do whatever it takes to get where you want to go.

# Congratulations!

## Rewards Week

You've successfully completed it through the (course name). Now it's time to celebrate and give yourself the reward you've been looking forward to. Treat yourself to a day spa. Go on a shopping spree. Take a mini-vacation and show off your new body. Even if you've not yet attained your ideal body, it's OK. I'm confident that you've followed this course as prescribed and you've significantly improved your physique and your health.

Once again, congratulations and take pride in the results you have achieved!

# TESTIMONIAL REQUEST

### We encourage you to share your success story!

### We are extremely interested in hearing your success story, as are countless others who face weight and fitness related issues.

You deserve to be recognized for your amazing achievements and by sharing your success with other, you are contributing to these individuals' sense of optimism and invoking in them the belief that they too can succeed.

Please take a few minutes to fill out the following profile and release form. You can also choose to send us your story via email to (enter email address) as long as you turn in the signed release form.

If you would like assistance in writing your testimonial, just ask! We are here to help. Simply ask your nutrition coach to set up a time to meet and reflect on your experience.

Thank you for taking the time to share. Once your testimonial is received, you will be presented with a token of our appreciation.

**Fat Loss Manifesto Testimonial**

Please describe the positive impact this course has had on your life, as well as your amazing results below.

_____ has my permission to quote from my comments and use my name and/or photographs for advertising, website and promotion. I waive the right to inspect or approve the photographs, promotional copy or printed matter that may be used in conjunction with, or as any part of advertising or promotion. I understand Fit Systems will not give or publish my address and/or phone number to anyone!

Signature: _____ Date: _____

Print Name: _____

## Appendices

~ Fitness Journal
~ Reflection Page

REFLECTION SHEET

**Session:**                                                    **Today's Date:**


Assimilation – Do I understand it? Do I have any questions?




What did I get out of this section?




**Action Plan:** List 3 ways I can use this information immediately:

**1.**

**2.**

**3.**




**Notes*Ideas* To-Do-List**




**Follow Up: 30 days later – Am I using it?**
**Why or why not?**

# FITNESS JOURNAL                                      **Date:**

My goal today:

| Supportive Nutrition: Factor 1 | Protein | Starchy Carb | Fibrous Carb | Cal ori es |
|---|---|---|---|---|
| Breakfast | | | | |
| Snack | | | | |
| Lunch | | | | |
| Snack | | | | |
| Dinner | | | | |
| Snack | | | | |

| Resistance Training: Factor 2 | Lbs/Reps | Lbs/Reps | Lbs/Reps |
|---|---|---|---|
| | / | / | / |
| | / | / | / |
| | / | / | / |
| | / | / | / |
| | / | / | / |
| | / | / | / |
| | / | / | / |
| | / | / | / |
| **Moderate Cardio: Factor 3** | NOTES: | | |

Type:

Minutes:

## Factor 4: My attitude today was:

Things I did today to be healthier:

Today, I Rewarded myself by:

I am most grateful for:

My biggest accomplishment today was:

My biggest setback today was:

# Fitness Tool Box

**A quick guide to jump start your fat loss journey**

The information in the packet is accurate. It is backed by science. Now it is up to you. You have to decide to make the change and live the life. Fitness is a lifestyle. It is a way of living. When you start living a fit lifestyle you will notice that your life will improve dramatically on many levels. It will improve socially, physically, and mentally. Your confidence will go up. You will live longer. You will look in the mirror and be proud of the face that is staring back at you for you will know you are doing all you can to live a healthy life, and that is a wonderful feeling.

And for everyone whom says that they don't have the time.......there are no excuses! I'm sure you make time for your favorite T.V. show or to go out to dinner. You just have to reorganize your priorities. Fitness should be one of your top priorities. Obesity rates are higher then ever and many health conditions follow. So if you feel it is selfish to take an hour a day four days a week for yourself to exercise, you shouldn't. Remember, your family, children, spouse, and friends all need you, but more importantly they NEED YOU HEALTHY!

Taking time for proper nutrition and exercise is not selfish- it is selfless for you are working to maintain your body to perform the tasks it requires and uphold relationships in your life for a longer time at a higher quality. If you ask a loved one if they would rather have all your time now and you'd be unhealthy and sickly in 15 years from now OR have moderate time with you and in 15 years continue to have you for you have taken care of your body and you are healthy.

 The answer is pretty clear. NO EXCUSES!!! Follow the guidelines set forth by your Fitness Professional as well as the information in this handbook and you will have no choice but to live a happier, leaner, healthier life.

# Healthy Habits Pyramid

Successful results can be achieved by simply replacing the habits that undermine your efforts with the new habits presented throughout this course.

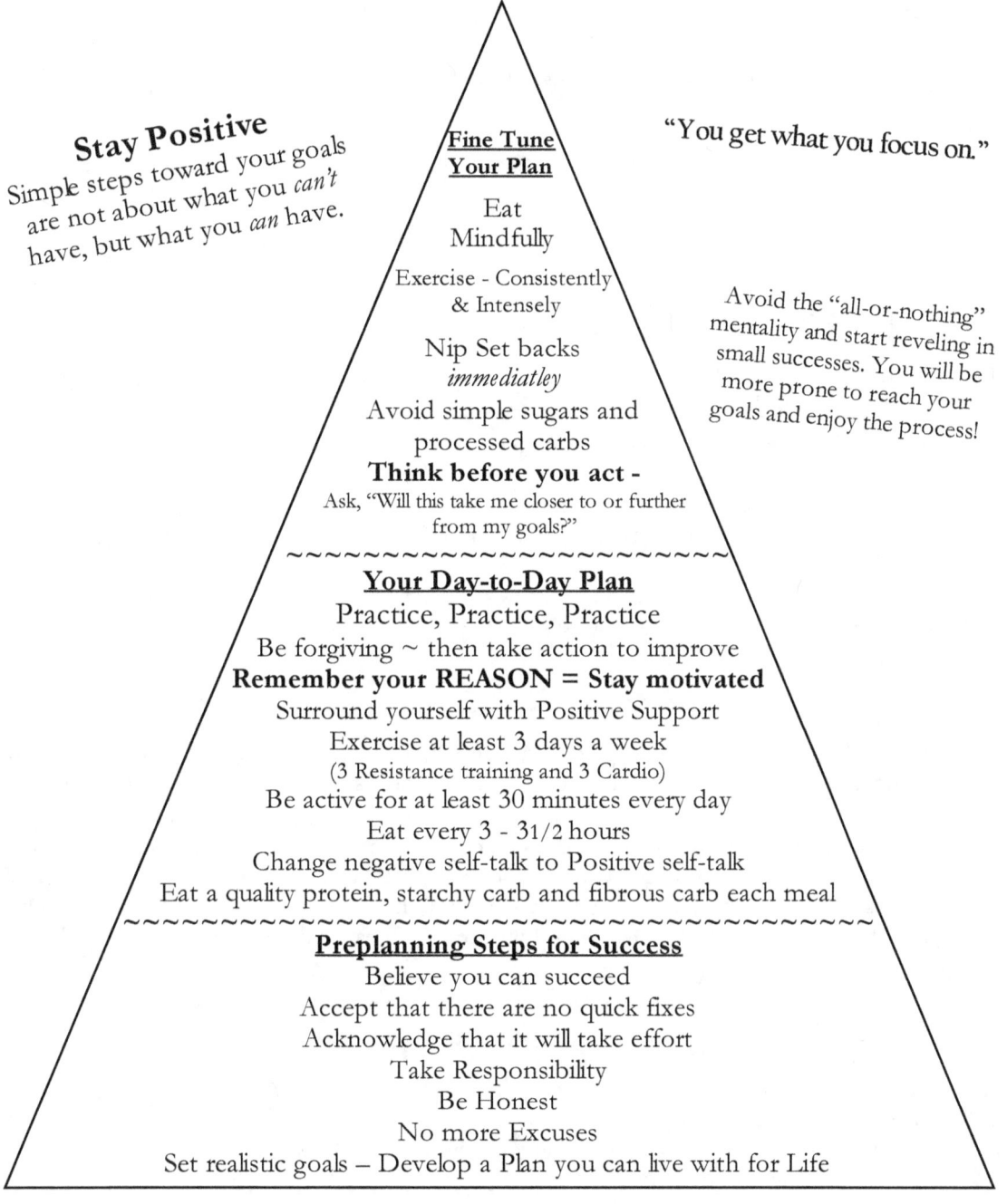

**Stay Positive**

Simple steps toward your goals are not about what you *can't* have, but what you *can* have.

"You get what you focus on."

**Fine Tune Your Plan**

Eat Mindfully

Exercise - Consistently & Intensely

Nip Set backs *immediatley*

Avoid simple sugars and processed carbs

**Think before you act -**

Ask, "Will this take me closer to or further from my goals?"

Avoid the "all-or-nothing" mentality and start reveling in small successes. You will be more prone to reach your goals and enjoy the process!

**Your Day-to-Day Plan**

Practice, Practice, Practice

Be forgiving ~ then take action to improve

**Remember your REASON = Stay motivated**

Surround yourself with Positive Support

Exercise at least 3 days a week

(3 Resistance training and 3 Cardio)

Be active for at least 30 minutes every day

Eat every 3 - 31/2 hours

Change negative self-talk to Positive self-talk

Eat a quality protein, starchy carb and fibrous carb each meal

**Preplanning Steps for Success**

Believe you can succeed

Accept that there are no quick fixes

Acknowledge that it will take effort

Take Responsibility

Be Honest

No more Excuses

Set realistic goals – Develop a Plan you can live with for Life

"Ability is what you're capable of doing. Motivation determines what you do.
Attitude determines how well you do it." - Lou Holtz

# The Solution Discovery Process

**Step One: Identify an area (areas) in need of a solution. Describe as clearly and completely as you can.** What is not working? Ask yourself what people, places, events, thoughts, or feelings make it difficult to:

> ➤ Control my eating/make better food choices?

> ➤ Be active today?

> ➤ Maintain a positive attitude?

**Step Two: Break each area down into smaller steps.** Think about each step one at a time so you are not overwhelmed. **Select the step(s) you wish to work on.**

You may discover only one step that you wish to address or you may have several. It is best to work on one or two at most at one time. Select the ones you will work on and focus your energy on dealing with them.

I WILL FOCUS ON:

**Step Three: Collect Ideas.** For the steps you've selected, identify some alternative ways to deal with them. The more ideas you identify, the easier it will be to find a solution that feels right for you.

Think of things that may have helped you deal with this challenge in the past. Start with the first step and write down possible ways in which you can address it. Maybe you can figure out a way to get to bed a little earlier? Maybe you can visit your family without having a meal? Maybe they can visit you instead at least some of the time? Perhaps you can learn to prepare simple meals at home and eat out less often?

Possible Resources:
~Ask your friends for ideas
~Talk to your Fitness Professional
~Read inspiring stories of those who have overcome similar situations
~Post a request for help on one of our BLOGS

Ask for additional ideas or advice from _____, personal training clients or other participants of this course.

BRAINSTORM IDEAS:

**Step Four: Decide What You will do**

Once you've identified several ways to deal with the issue at hand, select the idea you think will realistically work for you and what you are willing to do.

LIST your Plan of Action:

**Step Five: Do it!**

Use the idea you've selected to deal with your issue. If it does not work, try another. Sometimes it is a process of trial and error to find the solution that is best for you.

**Step Six: Evaluate Results**

Once you've dealt with the issue, evaluate how satisfied you were with the results.

- Were you able to make adjustments your eating habits?

- Were you able to follow through with workout plans?

- Were you able to deal with the problem to your satisfaction? If not, what would you do differently next time?

# Fat Loss Check List –
## 10 Reasons WHY you are not seeing results

1. You are eating TOO much. Even if you are carefully measuring and planning your main meals, extra calories can sneak in during snack. It is VERY common to significantly under-estimating the number of calories you are consuming on a daily basis. If you're not sure, write down everything you eat for one whole week.

2. You are not eating enough. You need to create a caloric deficit by reducing you calorie intake slightly. If you go too far below your maintenance calories, your body goes into starvation mode; sheds muscle and stores calories as fat, for a future energy source. Not eating enough supportive foods also lowers the amount of calories you burn….less thermic meals = less body fat burned.

3. You are not lifting weights – cardio burns calories but it doesn't boost your metabolism. Resistance training is *critical* to maintaining your muscle and tone. If you're not lifting weights while trying to lose body fat, you will lose muscle and tone and your metabolic rate will decrease causing you to burn fewer calories 24 hour-a-day!

4. You are simply not exercising anywhere near enough! You can only decrease your caloric intake so much before you start losing your fat burning muscle. The only other alternative is to increase calories out. VERY FEW people are successful at losing weight AND keeping it off without exercising almost everyday!! Make it a rule to be active at the very least 30 minutes a day.

If you're having trouble losing weight, 20 minutes of exercise three times a week isn't going to cut it! Most people who tell me they are *really serious* about losing weight are not willing to do what it takes to get where they want to be. If you're not willing to make exercise a *serious* priority in your life, your chances of succeeding at losing weight and keeping it off are VERY small!

5. Are you impatient? Are you looking for *instant* results? When it doesn't happen, you may give up. You HAVE to be resolved to the fact that it takes the integration of the Factors of Fat Loss and change WILL be slow yet steady! Try focusing on progress, not perfection

6. Are you any skipping meals? If so, do not expect to see results.  Skipping meals slows your metabolism causing body to store calories rather than burn them

7. Are you eating sugary foods or simple / refined carbohydrates?  White rice, white (non whole wheat) flour products, white pastas, soft drinks , sweetened drinks – like juice, and the hundreds of products that contain added sugar that's deceptively listed on ingredient lists with names like sucrose, high fructose corn syrup, etc. turns off the hormones responsible for releasing your body fat and instead turns ON the hormones that store fat.

8. How many alcoholic drinks do you have each week? Alcohol stimulates your appetite, slows your metabolism, and it's loaded with empty (sugar) calories!

9. Are you having fruits and/or vegetables EVERY time you eat? Are you taking your VGF+24 supplements every day?

10. Are you planning and preparing your meals ahead of time? If you have not planned your meals, you are more likely to cheat and find yourself off track.

As you can see, fat loss can be VERY difficult.......if you don't want it bad enough to do what it takes. If you really want to change, quit playing around with it. Get serious about it and make it an absolute, non-negotiable priority in your life... and it will happen!

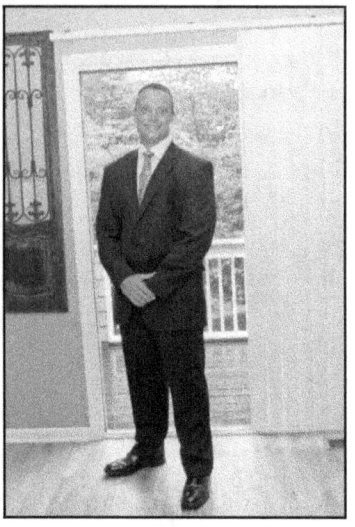

Referred to as one of the country's premier personal trainers, body transformation, and fat loss experts, Scott Hayward truly changes bodies and changes lives. As an author, lecturer, trainer, and educator, he is sought out by those looking to transform their bodies and ultimately transform their lives.

Scott, who holds numerous degrees and certifications, is the author of; "Absession...America's Guide to Ultimate 6 Pack Abs," as well as numerous articles on Anatomy, Physiology, Energy Metabolism, and Exercise Science. His seminars, lectures and workshops on fat loss, weight loss, and body transformation techniques have transformed thousands of lives.

Scott is the consulting exercise physiologist for a fitness product development company, which has several exciting pieces of fitness equipment slated for release in the near future.

Scott and his training techniques were the 2 term official trainer for the Miss Pennsylvania USA Pageant, and has provided training for; NFL, NCAA, NBA and MLS Players. Scott has also been sought out to train Hollywood movie stars, daytime television stars and music icons.

Scott owned and operated an 8,000 square foot Personal Training Facility. He was the fitness director for a 3,000 member health and fitness facility, participated in and coached college athletics and was an adjunct professor for several nationally accredited personal training certifications.

Scott is married to Jennifer Lynn Hayward and they reside in the Philadelphia region with their Siberian Husky named Zoey. Together they have formed Fit for Faith Ministries. Fit for Faith Ministries is a Christian Fitness Ministry which is dedicated to educating, inspiring and empowering people to become better stewards of the body God has given them. Fit for Faith Ministry conducts fat loss seminars and body transformation programs for churches throughout the region.

Check out Fit for Faith on the web at www.fitforfaithministries.com

www.ingramcontent.com/pod-product-compliance
Lightning Source LLC
Chambersburg PA
CBHW080432290526
45791CB00008BA/2466

* 9 7 8 1 4 9 4 4 3 4 2 1 2 *